QUEER MINDS

from the author

The Trans Guide to Mental Health and Wellbeing
Katy Lees
ISBN 978 1 78775 526 0
eISBN 978 1 78775 527 7

of related interest

The Queer Mental Health Workbook
A Creative Self-Help Guide Using CBT, CFT and DBT
Dr Brendan J Dunlop
ISBN 978 1 83997 107 5
eISBN 978 1 83997 108 2

The Trans Self Care Workbook
A Coloring Book and Journal for Trans and Non-Binary People
Theo Lorenz
ISBN 978 1 78775 343 3
eISBN 978 1 78775 344 0

The Anxiety Book for Trans People
How to Conquer Your Dysphoria, Worry Less and Find Joy
Freiya Benson
ISBN 978 1 78775 223 8
eISBN 978 1 78775 224 5

The Autistic Trans Guide to Life
Yenn Purkis and Wenn Lawson
Foreword by Dr Emma Goodall
ISBN 978 1 78775 391 4
eISBN 978 1 78775 392 1

Queer Minds

*LGBTQ+ Therapists and Advocates
on Mental Health, Neurodivergence,
and the Things That Help*

KATY LEES

Jessica Kingsley Publishers
London and Philadelphia

First published in Great Britain in 2026 by Jessica Kingsley Publishers
An imprint of John Murray Press

1

A CIP catalogue record for this title is available from the
British Library and the Library of Congress.

ISBN 978 1 80501 181 1
eISBN 978 1 80501 182 8

Printed and bound in Great Britain by Clays Ltd

Jessica Kingsley Publishers' policy is to use papers that are
natural, renewable and recyclable products and made from wood
grown in sustainable forests. The logging and manufacturing
processes are expected to conform to the environmental
regulations of the country of origin.

Jessica Kingsley Publishers
Carmelite House
50 Victoria Embankment
London EC4Y 0DZ

www.jkp.com

John Murray Press
Part of Hodder & Stoughton Ltd
An Hachette Company

The authorised representative in the EEA is Hachette Ireland,
8 Castlecourt Centre, Dublin 15, D15 XTP3, Ireland (email: info@hbgi.ie)

For Lucy, whose heart I carry in my heart.

Contents

Acknowledgements

Thanks and everlasting love to all of the *Queer Minds* interview collaborators – Gem, Emily, Emma, LJ, Viv, Rae, Jess, Rory, Lucy, Sage, Kai, Sorel, and Stef. You are all amazing, and none of this exists without you.

Thanks and congratulations to everyone at Jessica Kingsley Publishers, especially Jane Evans, Laura Dignum-Smith, Carys Homer, Adam Peacock, Helen Kemp, Rosamund Bird, and Alex DiFrancesco, who each offered help and support through the creation of this book. We did it!

Thanks and well wishes to Andrew James, the editor who got me through writing my first published book, *The Trans Guide to Mental Health and Well-Being*, and the person who originally invited me to write *Queer Minds*. Your belief in me has been life changing.

Thanks and admiration to Juno Roche, whose unmissable book *Queer Sex* was one of the central inspirations for *Queer Minds*. Your wisdom, bravery, and openness have made such a difference to queer minds everywhere.

Last, but not least, thanks again to Lucy, this second time for the reminders to hydrate, the enthusiastic encouragement, the kind and firm suggestion that I take breaks, and everything else you gave me while I worked on this project. I love you!

Introduction

Why queer minds?

More people than ever are coming out as queer: 1.5 million people in England and Wales alone identify as LGB+ (Roskams, 2023), and approximately 600,000 people in the United Kingdom identify as trans and/or non-binary (Stonewall, 2021). Globally, just under 10% of the population identify as part of the LGBTQ2SA+ community (Jackson, 2023), which is over 700 million people worldwide. While increasing numbers of LGBTQ+ people are coming out (Jones, 2022; Sharfman and Cobb, 2023; Pappy, 2024), and there is more queer visibility than ever (Flores, 2021; Jackson, 2023), there is also a lasting misunderstanding of who queer people are and how they think. For example, 90% of trans and/or non-binary people have been – inaccurately – told they were 'not normal' (McNeil *et al.*, 2012), and most report that their mental health needs are not currently being met (Watkinson *et al.*, 2024). Labelling LGBTQ+ communities as 'mentally ill' has long been a tactic of oppression, and it was only in 2019 that the World Health Organization (WHO) stopped categorizing transness as a 'mental disorder' (Haynes, 2019).

Clearly there's an issue here, and it's beyond time that more attention is paid to how queer people think, feel, and experience the world. There are so many questions to consider when it comes to queer minds! What do we think about, dream about, and connect to? What helps us, or holds us down? What kind of support do we need to take care of our minds? How do we learn, heal, and love?

These are important questions for the LGBTQ+ community, for the allistic people (that is, people who are allosexual, cisgender, and heterosexual) who love us, and for the people who are called to help us look after our bodies and minds. As a non-binary and queer psychotherapist myself, I've seen how common and varied issues around mental health and neurodiversity often are for queer people. All of my current therapy clients are LGBTQ+ in some way, and the vast majority are trans and/or non-binary. Research suggests that LGBTQ+ people have higher rates of depression (Cai *et al.*, 2024), disordered eating (Parker and Harriger, 2020), post-traumatic stress (Keating and Muller, 2019), and much more, due to our experiences of oppression and minority stress (Meyer, 2003; Lefevor *et al.*, 2019). There's also evidence that neurodivergent people are more likely than allocishet people to identify as LGBTQ+ (Strang *et al.*, 2014; Dewinter, De Graaf, and Begeer, 2017; George and Stokes, 2018; Warrier *et al.*, 2020; Mangen, 2023), which means queer people are more likely to be autistic, ADHD, OCD, dyspraxic, dyscalculic, dyslexic, or any another natural human variation that means the way they process information is not considered typical in society, and this is something I definitely see in the majority of my clients, as well as myself. My LGBTQ+ therapy clients also tend to be in 'non-normative' relationships, as well as prioritizing 'found families' and built communities, all of which is very normal and enriching but which is often misunderstood and pathologized by mental health practitioners who aren't in the know.

As a neurodivergent trauma survivor and user of mental health services, too, I've seen first-hand how misunderstood LGBTQ+ people can be in mental health spaces, and how important queer-affirming mental health practices are. Queer minds deserve a level of understanding that we don't always get but which can feel like coming home when we do. Queer mental health workers are often missed and underrepresented in the profession, too (Holmberg, Martin, and Lunn, 2022; Bizzeth and Beagan, 2023; Chamlou, 2024), which only decreases the chances that queer mental health clients will find someone who 'gets it'. Knowing that we are understood, and being able to feel that consistently and deeply, is so important for our mental and emotional health, and it is something that everyone deserves.

Queer mental health is obviously an important topic, and queer voices need to be heard on the subject. My experience is that queer minds are often at the forefront of mental health issues on all sides, navigating the psychiatric system, therapy, community care, self-care, hardship, healing, and more – but, in my experience, this is so rarely talked about openly and broadly. I have so often had to dive deeply to find any accessible and affirming words from queer mental health and neurodiversity experts speaking directly to queer people. Queer minds are inherently interesting, and we have a lot to contribute in all areas of mental health and neurodivergence.

With this collection of interviews, I wanted to examine a broad and interesting cross-section of queer life with reflections on mental health and neurodiversity at the centre. I hoped to learn more from, and connect with, as many queer experts as possible, and I wanted to include as many different kinds of expertise as possible from as many different ways of being as I could. I wanted to centre the things that people have found helpful, too, and to explore the ways that LGBTQ+ individuals and communities can find comfort, change, and connection. I've done this by conducting a series of interviews with LGBTQ+ therapists, advocates, and more, all of whom have unique insights into different kinds of queer minds. I'm excited to share their incredible words with you!

An introduction to me, the interviewer

I am Katy Lees (they/them), a person-centred psychotherapist with expertise in queer mental health and wellness. I've been working in mental health since 2007, and I've been a mental health service user for longer. My work in mental health has taken place in a varied number of settings and I'm now working in a settled private psychotherapy practice that prioritizes LGBTQ+ experiences. It's imperative for both me and my clients that I run my practice in a person-centred, anti-racist, anti-oppressive, neurodiversity affirming, queer knowledgeable way that is as accessible as I can make it, and I work to bring those principles to this book, too.

As well as working closely with LGBTQ+ clients, I'm also queer and non-binary, and I've been out as some flavour of queer for about as long as I've been working in mental health. Queerness aside, I am a white, neurodivergent, disabled, working class, mid fat, English person in my 30s, and these aspects of privilege and oppression are always a part of my work, including these interviews, whether intentionally or not.

My use of the term 'queer'

I've used the term 'queer' throughout this book as a reclaimed term to mean 'a sexuality and/or gender identity that lies along a broad spectrum of non-straight and non-cisgender normativity'. 'Queer' has been used neutrally – and positively – as both an individual descriptor of gender and attraction, and as a community-based description of shared non-allocishet experience, for a long time; and it's with this benign and radical spirit that I use the term 'queer' to describe my book collaborators, my community, this book, and myself.

The interview process

In the early days of working on this book, I got to spend a couple of really fun days doing some blue-sky thinking about the interesting queer people in my life that might want to participate in this project. I'm fortunate to know many amazing LGBTQ+ people with varied insights into how queer minds work. I know some of these experts personally, and some through social media or professional peripheries, and I feel extremely thankful that so many cool people trusted me with their thoughts, feelings, and experiences for this book. Every interviewee here was chosen because I knew their perspective would be interesting in a unique way, and because they had inspired me in some way in my therapy work or my personal growth as a queer person. I wanted to include as many different queer perspectives here from all kinds of personal accounts, with QTBIPOC, transfeminine, disabled, fat, and working class perspectives taking priority.

At each stage of the process I tried my best to be upfront that contributors could be as open or as anonymous as felt comfortable through each stage of the process. I was careful to let everyone know they could answer – or not answer – any question without judgement, and also that they could ignore all of my questions and go completely off road with the interview if they wanted. I offered every contributor a small payment, a skill trade, and/or a donation to their fund of choice in return for their interview, and I wish I could have offered much more.

I sent the interviewees their proposed interview questions before the interview so they could have time to think about their answers, correct any of my assumptions in the offered questions, and suggest anything they really wanted to talk about ahead of time. I had hoped that sharing the questions in advance would make things more accessible for my interviewees – I know I'm less anxious about interviews if I have time to prepare my answers. I asked people to only answer the questions that felt comfortable, and I tried to make this clear in both the emailed questions and in the face-to-face interview. Everybody's first official interview question was the same – 'Tell me about yourself!'

All of the interviews were completed virtually over video call. I edited the transcripts for clarity – mostly taking out any 'um's and 'hmmm's – while working to keep the content and context intact. Everyone received a copy of their transcript to check through, with the invitation to add, delete, change, clarify, or withdraw anything. If any words were changed for clarity or to protect confidential identities, it was always with my interviewee's consent. In the transcripts, I've used ( ) to indicate an aside from me to add context, and [ ] to add tone or expression.

All of these interviews happened in 2023–2024, so all of these thoughts were shared under a backdrop of several genocides worldwide, increasingly unfunded mental health care in all areas, racist rioting in the UK, and the continued effects of the covid-19 pandemic. The impact of these events ripples through these accounts of queerness and in my own interviewing.

Content advisory

This is a book detailing LGBTQ+ people's lived experiences of mental health and neurodiversity. There's a lot of joy, hope, and community in this book, and there are also potentially difficult topics discussed here. Please be advised that the people in this book talk about facing both general and individual instances of discrimination against LGBTQ+ people, including transphobia, homophobia, biphobia, and more. There is also discussion of some highly traumatic elements of queerphobia and mental health discrimination, including bullying, conversion therapy, and being sectioned. Different kinds of discrimination are discussed, including experiences of racism, ableism, and fatphobia. Please take care of yourself if you find yourself affected, and check out the resources at the end of each chapter.

Radical Community Care with Sage Stephanou

An introduction to Sage

Sage Stephanou (they/them) is a community facilitator, an anti-oppressive consultant, an abolitionist educator, a clinical supervisor to therapists, and one of the principal people behind the Radical Therapist Network. They're a non-binary, queer, working class, disabled, mixed heritage person whose work centres transformative justice, decolonial therapeutic work, and collective care.

I've followed Sage's work for some time now through the Radical Therapy Network, a UK-based community aiming to dismantle white supremacy in therapeutic spaces and in general. The importance of therapeutic communities like the Radical Therapist Network has only become clearer during my time as a therapist. This book was written – and my therapeutic career has been fostered – during a run of persistent, escalating violence against minoritized people around the world in places like Palestine (Oxfam International, 2024), Ukraine (Walton, 2022), Sudan (Human Rights Watch, 2024), Congo (UNICEF, 2021), the USA (McKinley, 2024; Meckler, Natanson, and Harden, 2024), and the UK (Goodier, 2023; White, 2024). Western therapy training is overwhelmingly white and allocishet in terms of its foundations (Naughton and Tudor, 2017), its training models and trainers (Ellis and Cooper, 2013; Haskins *et al.*, 2013; McKenzie-Mavinga, 2007), and the people who can make their way through training (Lin, Stamm, and Christidis, 2018), something I've unfortunately seen play out in my own training and therapeutic communities. The colonial legacy this creates at the centre of Western mental health care is one that has led to harmful allocisheteronormativity in therapeutic spaces (Neves, 2023; Moses and Cole, 2023).

I was excited to talk to Sage because I knew they would have excellent insights to share, especially around decolonizing therapeutic spaces, the overwhelming whiteness of therapy training institutes, and supporting queer people of colour as mental health practitioners and service users. I've followed their work for a long time while I've worked to end white supremacy in my queer therapy practice and my life, and I admire everything about them that they've chosen to share.

Sage's interview

Sage: Thank you for inviting me here. It feels really lovely to have been asked. I'm really excited about your book, and its potential, and the juiciness of it.

Katy: Me, too! You were one of the first people that I thought of to talk to. Thank you for being here. Do you want to tell me a bit about yourself?

Sage: A bit about myself? I am quite a shy person, and often really rubbish at saying a bit about myself, so that also feels like part of myself. So, I'm gonna start there!

I am, by profession, an art psychotherapist, and I've also done my Bachelor of Arts training in creative expressive therapies. I'm a facilitator, but on the whole I like to describe myself as a community worker. I'm a person that uses the skills I've learned to hold spaces in community for community, and that is often support-based spaces, embodied healing spaces, and experiential learning spaces. I'm also a clinical supervisor to therapists, and organizations with aligned values, as well as providing consultation. I'm an educator as well; having lectured within the academy, I fell in love with being able to provide and receive education in a reciprocal way. And so a lot of my work, especially in the Radical Therapist Network, is to provide anti-colonial learning spaces for therapists and healers who hold privileged, dominant identities in the field.

Katy: That's really cool! What is it like to be a queer therapist, or a queer mental health professional, in England right now?

Sage: Thank you for this question. I don't think I can talk about queerness without talking about my trans experience, and I can't talk about being trans without also talking about my experiences of being a mixed heritage person of the Global Majority. I would also need to talk about familial experiences of forced migration, colonialism, war, intergenerational trauma, and my own personal lived experience of poverty, homelessness, and liminality. So for me to talk about myself as a queer therapist I would need to honour my personal narrative as a London-born, working class, mixed heritage, disabled, non-binary person residing in Nottingham. And that's complex, because it doesn't fit the normative experience of traditional Western therapists. That is often the experience of multiply marginalized therapists.

So, in short, what is it to be a queer therapist as a multiply marginalized person? I would say that it's a challenge, and it's lonely – but outside of practising as a therapist, and in community, it's nourishing and it's reciprocal. It's creative, it's joyful. For me there's a really vast difference in my experience of practising as a therapist

– as a queer therapist – in the traditional sense, and that being a battle, and then the experience of being a queer therapist who is a community worker, where that is a much more validating, holding experience.

Katy: That sounds so much more fulfilling for everyone.

Sage: Absolutely.

In the questions you sent in advance, you asked a really beautiful question: 'What do you wish more therapists would work on in their practice and outside of their practice to help their clients?' I want to follow on from what I was saying around the white experience being the dominant narrative.

I think one of the things that I've been really disheartened by within the white queer therapist community, so to speak, is complicity through silence. I've been thinking about how having a shared marginalized identity doesn't necessarily equate to shared solidarity. I'm known for talking a lot about whiteness and white supremacy but that's because, as a therapist working within these systems, I can't not talk about whiteness as an embodiment of white supremacy culture, and how queerness doesn't exempt white therapists from enacting harm either explicitly, through their actions in the therapy room, or implicitly, through their silence within institutions or politically.

I think Palestine is a really heart-wrenching example of this. Since 7 October 2023, there's been complete silence from prominent therapy organizations who are yet to speak out against the settler colonial imperial violence that's ongoing. With the ongoing genocide in Palestine, as of today, it's 101 days and 75 years of ongoing bombing and ethnic cleansing, which has led to over 30,000 deaths (at the time this book was published; since then many more days and many more deaths have occurred). This monumental moment in history, the monumental violence that is happening, I can't – I can't, in my heart – hold the weight of how many therapists, in particular, aren't saying anything. As Ericka Hart says, 'Your queerness does not absolve your racism' (Hart, 2023).

So many of my teachers have been Black women – Black, gender non-conforming women in particular – and that's how I position a lot of my thinking and practice. When many white queer people were collectively speaking out against this genocide, a prominent discourse has been – as you, I'm sure, have already heard – 'Palestinians are homophobic, you'd get killed for being queer there.' As if queer Palestinians don't exist, as if that should be a justification for mass murder, as if European colonizers haven't attempted to erase queer people of colour in colonized cultures for hundreds of years as part of the colonial project that benefits our current white supremacist society today.

I talk about that, because it's those white supremacist systems and cultures that we are educated within as therapists, including queer therapists. We need to understand that universities and academies in the UK are built on the profits of the transatlantic slave trade, and that our Western theories are created by racist patriarchal European men. The foundations of Western therapy are founded on white supremacist ideology. Therefore, how can we curate healing conditions within the four walls of the master's house?

My work, as a multiply marginalized community worker who also has proximity to whiteness, is to constantly disrupt white supremacy in every facet of this work, because healing justice cannot be nurtured under oppressive conditions, even if those conditions were created or maintained by well-meaning therapists.

Katy: I'm really hearing that and thinking about how I obviously have to sit with myself and keep doing the work. I've learned recently that some trans people I had respected are Zionists. It really shocked me. I had to sit with myself and be like, 'Why am I shocked that these white queer people want to uphold colonization?' This shouldn't have shocked me.

Sage: Thank you for sharing that with me. I'm really sorry that that's been your experience.

I think, as a community, we have to hold each other accountable. I don't mean that in a punitive sense, in the way that that's often co-opted, but how can we hold space together within our more privileged aspects of identity to unlearn and be with discomfort around those things? I'm not necessarily suggesting that's what you should have done with the people you had respected before but, just as a whole, how can we hold space together to be with that discomfort? Because, otherwise, who are we expecting to do that work? And that, I think, especially needs to happen within more marginalized communities like queer communities, because that's also where harm can become compounded, right?

Katy: Yeah, absolutely. Thank you for sharing. What is it like, facilitating queer communities?

Sage: Interestingly, my experience of facilitating for queer community actually hasn't always been that positive. It's because of the dominant white experience – especially where I'm living in the East Midlands, it's predominantly white. That meant that I was organizing community spaces that were attended by predominantly white queers. What I noticed was, when racist experiences did come up within the queer community by white people, the more marginalized Black and brown individuals were then excluded and had to leave those spaces. My attempts to call out and address that racism resulted in backlash. There's been a consistent theme, unfortunately, of racism within the queer community, which I think circles back to how we hold each other accountable.

However, more widely, when I practise as a facilitator where it's not centring one aspect of identity, that has often felt nurturing because it's ended up being more peer led and held in a way that diffuses power relations and power dynamics. It starts with this idea of me being the facilitator, and then the group hierarchy starts to flatten when working in peer-led ways.

Katy: That sounds really interesting and so much better. This feeds into another of my questions – what does radical therapy mean to you, and how do you practise it?

Sage: Sometimes people ask me, 'Do radical takes on therapy mean we should abolish therapy? What else is there if we take therapy away?' I think that is a very all or nothing approach, which is incredibly binary, and therefore reduces our capacity to imagine alternative possibilities.

For example, I think of the Black Panthers (a Black power organization based in the USA and UK in the 1960s–1980s), who lived and worked in community to create healthy ways of life that don't rely on policing and abolition in that context. That looked like providing breakfast for children every day, providing health care, providing education and community protection. For me, that's an example of abolishing systems of surveillance, racism, and state violence, which therapy is actively complicit and enmeshed with.

To contextualize this a bit more, an example of that enmeshment as therapists is a requirement (in the UK) to undertake the Prevent duty training, which, as I'm sure you know, is a racist and Islamophobic policy that allegedly safeguards vulnerable people from extremism and radicalization. In practice, what that looks like is therapists working within systems, such as schools and hospitals, and referring racialized clients to the government, creating exposure to state surveillance, criminalization, and further harm. This is one aspect of how therapists criminalize distress.

An alternative would look like divesting from the systems of violence, which often means losing power. If we're contracted to undertake Prevent training in our workplace, we may have to leave those institutions. In that same vein, I have also been reported to the Department of Education as an anti-white extremist.

Katy: Hell yeah!

Sage: [Sage laughs] I've actually put that on the top of my CV! [Both laugh] 'Sage Stephanou, Anti-White Extremist!' I was actually reported for my anti-racist work within the Radical Therapist Network. I think that is the power that we have, to be willing to give up privilege and be willing to face the repercussions, especially if we hold power. In my case, that would be my proximity to whiteness as a mixed heritage person.

When we look at models of community care that prioritize community-led mental health responses and support that don't rely on the police, and are underpinned by creating infrastructure that is holistic, we broaden our definition of what therapy can be and what liberation and healing justice can look like. We need abolitionist, disability justice-led community work that understands that good health isn't possible without access to safe housing, to safe and free health care, to food, to safe and nourishing community connection, to joy.

We can't provide effective therapy to a hungry child who's just left their cold house that is infested with mould and is constantly unwell and is, therefore, having to miss school often – and guess what happens when those kids keep missing school? Punishment. Exclusion. Then that child is led onto a path of the school-to-prison pipeline. So we can see how easy it becomes for the state to punish and criminalize our racialized and disabled children and families. This is what it means to find alternatives to the Western therapy as we know it, and practise it, and have been recruited to work within it.

Healing justice can never coexist along State provision. We must divest, so our energy can be poured into autonomous community wells. This supports an anti-capitalist, anti-colonial practice that thrives on mutuality and interdependence. These institutions, and the State, really rely on individuals who deeply love and care about their work to the point of burnout. It's in contrast to this community care, which understands that sustainability requires many hands, and actively rejects individualistic, paternalistic, white saviourism, which is what therapy is based on in the West.

To give an example of how this is actually practised, there's a report called *Defund the Police – Invest in Community Care: A Guide to Alternative Mental Health Responses.* It's a really beautiful report – I really recommend reading it. It outlines two case studies where they have successfully implemented community initiatives that practise disability justice and peer-led alternatives. They are called CAT-911 and Fireweed Collective, both based in the States, and they're both self-sufficient in offering models that address conflict resolution, mental health crises, police violence, sexual violence, domestic violence, and peer-led support spaces. When we talk about what abolition in therapy can look like, we're seeing it happening in practice in the community and, for me, that's a little bit of what my facilitation of work looks like now, rather than practising as a therapist.

Katy: That sounds so important. I'm excited to check out those resources. It's so nice to hear that this is out there. I mean, I know and believe that things like this are working out there, but it's nice that there's so much concrete evidence of the different ways that this is done well.

Sage: It's very cool! And it's cool that it's not just one project, but so many ongoing acts and moments as well. There's so much evidence of how we can practise that in an everyday way and divest from harmful practices in small, everyday doses.

Katy: There's so much chance for real connection. What helps you to feel connected when things feel hard?

Sage: I really love and appreciate that question, because I think that is part and parcel of the work.

Mariame Kaba is an African American woman who is a prison abolitionist, and she famously wrote that 'hope is a discipline' (Kaba, 2021, p.47). That is a mantra that I often return to, to support my work and when I feel worn down. It's something I think about when I'm moving towards hopelessness, usually because I'm exhausted, in pain, feeling isolated, feeling angry. When I'm in that place – emotionally, spiritually, psychologically – I try to turn and look towards what my peers and community are engaging in, and I always reflect back to what my ancestors have endured, and I enter the movements that have existed and that we are currently building upon. I connect to all of those things and move away from a nihilistic state of hopelessness – because that hopelessness is also a function of white supremacist culture, to individualize pain and to become insular. For my pain to be individualized is so easy to do as a disabled person who lives by themself. When I'm in pain I'm often in pain by myself, and I can get very stuck in my head, and I have to resist that pull to feel sorry for myself and keep looking outwards. I remind myself that I also need to ask for help.

I've spoken a little bit about moving away from individualistic practices and white saviourist practices as therapists. I've also mentioned reciprocity a few times, in particular in regards to facilitation, and I had to learn through the process of practising community care to also be visibly vulnerable. And that fucking sucks! And I hate it! And it's also been one of the most beautiful, loving, healing experiences. It's something I have to practise often, because I am marginalized, within my different identities.

I think that also links, for me, into what it means to be an educator. To be an educator is also to learn to receive care, and to break down those positions of facilitator, group, therapist, client, to really practise a more egalitarian partnership. That's what helps me feel connected – to be part of the struggle, but also to be part of the healing. It's not binary, and we have to share our power in order to create the change we want to see.

Katy: That sounds like such a difficult and lovely experience for all of you in the community.

Sage: Absolutely. When I talk about community, I think that also means a lot of different things. I think for lots of queer therapists, and multiply marginalized therapists, we're often working in isolation, and there isn't necessarily a fixed local community. I think the pandemic has propelled that, actually. I work from home because of the pandemic, in part, and so I'm often not physically seeing anyone and I'm working on a screen. That has also meant that I've been able to connect internationally with people – you know, we're able to have *this* conversation because of the internet! I think that's also really wonderful. You were saying that you also work from home and remotely?

Katy: Yeah! I started working remotely because of the pandemic, but also because of chronic health stuff, and because I'm a carer, and because of my increasing understanding of my own neurodiversity. It's helped me to find a different kind of community for me, which has been difficult and essential.

Sage: In what ways do you feel like it's been difficult and essential?

Katy: I feel like community has always been quite difficult for me, especially because I've spent a lot of time living in places in the northeast of England where diversity is hidden and excluded, unfortunately. It's been difficult to find not just people like me – who are queer and trans and neurodivergent and chronically ill and anti-diet and disabled – but also people who aren't like me – like people of colour.

I did manage to find myself a nice little local queer community, actually, but then when the pandemic happened – I mean, it's still happening, but – that wasn't around anymore. Trying to find that online very much felt like starting again. I had to fight the urge to be isolated, to withdraw into myself with how painful it was to start again. As you say, though, it's been really fulfilling to find different kinds of community, online and over Zoom – like in this interview! It's been amazing to find different kinds of peers, and to widen my idea of who my peers are.

Sage: Who would you have initially thought your peers were?

Katy: I thought of my peers as the therapists I had trained with as a student. I trained at a very white institution – or it was when I trained there, I'm not sure now. Most of the trainees and trainers were white, cis, and straight. They were as much 'my community' as I could find in that arena.

Being able to find more therapists that I can interact with – in online training, in remote supervision, in mental health and activist social spaces online – has been everything. I've been able to look for paid training that is led by, for example, Black trans women online. I've been really trying to prioritize reading mental health books written by people of colour. I've been trying to learn from them how white, allocishet ideas of how we 'should' be doing therapy, and how we should be looking at things like attachment theory, are built on white violence. I've been trying to learn and unlearn. It's been good! It's been fulfilling. I'm glad that I found those people. I'm glad that I'm still finding these people.

Sage: Thank you for sharing that. It sounds like it's also been really hard work to find that for yourself.

Katy: At the beginning it was hard work because I didn't know where to look. The more people that I find, the more training I do, and the more books I read, it's really snowballed. I feel like I'm really finding good people now.

Sage: I'm really glad to hear that! That makes me feel really happy!

Katy: Speaking of good spaces, I'm really interested in what it was like to set up the Radical Therapist Network (RTN)?

Sage: It was an accident, at first. It wasn't set up with the intention to become what it is today. It was set up in response to experiences of violence, racism, and anti-Blackness in universities. That led me to a place of hopelessness, and then to a place of rage. It was that rage that led me to put a call out across social media to therapists who might also identify as sharing radical politics, and it's built from there quite organically.

I still feel quite surprised at how many therapists have shown up, and continue to show up, to find ways to organize. That, in part, was aided by the pandemic moving us online. It has also, therefore, enabled us to create much more accessible work, because it's cut out barriers such as a lot of work being London-centred. That's enabled connection across the UK and internationally.

It's been a really beautiful experience, but it's also been a difficult experience, because it has meant having to do a lot of unlearning work with therapists, and that has been incredibly fulfilling but also somatically exhausting and spiritually depleting. The direction that we're moving in is working out how to continue to offer and co-create work that is more sustainable.

The work that RTN does is to provide decolonial, anti-colonial learning spaces and unlearning spaces. So, people who are white, middle class, traditionally trained therapists within the UK can come and be held gently and firmly accountable, while providing resources to unlearn and relearn what community care can look like, and how to shift therapy practice in a more radical direction. The work that we do at the Radical Therapist Network is to offer experiential, embodied group work, because colonization means really processing how white supremacy and colonialism is deeply embedded into our bodies. That has to be made sense of, and processed, so that we don't continue to enact that violence within the therapy room. We also provide community care by offering peer support spaces, and that comes in the form of support groups, peer-led support groups, and peer supervision, but also offering more widely supportive spaces that are restorative for community. Most recently, that has been in response to the genocide in Palestine. This work is becoming more and more embedded in community and modelling what alternative therapies can look like through our own praxis.

Katy: That's such important work. You were saying that part of this work is about making things more accessible for people in the network, like holding sessions online. How do you make your therapeutic practices and your facilitation more accessible for you? How do you look after yourself through what must be important, exhausting work?

Sage: Thank you for that question. That feels really important.

I consistently have to resist the pull – the inner temptation, the demands from others – to work. I have to resist my internal dialogue when I'm sick, that says, 'You should be working. You should be doing something. Your worth is intrinsically tied to production and output.' I remind myself constantly that resting, reluctantly or not, is part of modelling community care, because if I am sick as a person in community, I am not able to provide the same depth of care work in an ethical and safe way. I've had to reframe what work looks like for me as a chronically ill disabled person, where I can't work nine to five.

Part of that reframing has been understanding that rest is part of the work so, when I am resting, I am working. That's also a really frustrating experience because sometimes, when I'm resting, I want to be able to read a book. I want to be able to have a conversation. I want to be able to think – and, when you're sick, you can't necessarily do these things. And so resting actually feels incredibly political, because it's not necessarily enjoyable. It's often quite a lonely experience, as I'm sure you might resonate with.

Katy: For sure.

Sage: So part of learning to rest has also been, again, learning to be vulnerable. That has enabled me to connect with other disabled folks online, which has meant being able to have space to be seen and connect on much deeper levels. A lot of my healing and learning have come from other disabled people of the Global Majority, where that experience of disability is informed by intergenerational trauma and colonial legacies. I can't separate how violence towards land also means violence towards the body, and what is carried in our bodies. My understanding of how to rest with that knowledge of that history, which is located in my body, and that practice of rest also then honours my ancestors and enables me to connect and heal in a much more spiritual way than capitalist ideas of self-care can ever understand.

I'm moving away from consumerist, capitalist ideas of what self-care and rest look like. I'm moving back towards collective and community care as self-care. How I look after myself impacts the work that we can do.

Katy: How do you think therapy can be a cause for radical decolonial justice? I guess we've already addressed that it pretty much fails to do this...

Sage: Within Western practices, I think so, yeah, but outside of that, so many alternatives exist to practise. Outside of that, there is hope.

Katy's post-interview thoughts

As expected, Sage was a delight to listen to and share with, and I left this interview carrying a renewed hopefulness. As we spoke about community care as self-care – and vice versa – I was reminded of the endless ways we can be together as queer people.

Sage also offered an important reminder to reconnect with my hope that queer people can survive and thrive. So often systems of oppression work to make us feel hopeless, powerless, and alone, and this conversation with Sage was a powerful reminder that therapists – particularly white therapists, like me – can be involved in calling people in towards accountability while also resisting our inner cops.

I also left with renewed questions about my therapeutic work, which maybe you can ask yourself, too, if you hold some societal power. How am I going to hold that hopeful space of resistance going forward – with myself, with my clients, with other therapists, with my queer community at large – to learn from the discomfort that comes with recognizing and destroying my privilege? How am I supporting oppressed people, particularly LGBTQ+ people of the Global Majority, in remaining in safe communities and creating their own power? How am I participating in the oppression of others and myself?

If you'd like to know more

Radical Therapist Network. Sage is the founder and co-director of the Radical Therapist Network, an essential community-based learning and support network working to support therapists to dismantle, unlearn, and heal from white supremacy and colonialism. www.radicaltherapistnetwork.com

Sister Outsider: Essays and Speeches, by Audre Lorde, 1984. A seminal collection of work with a sharp eye towards ending marginalization and building community, including the essay 'The Master's Tools Will Never Dismantle the Master's House', which was referenced by Sage in their interview.

We Do This 'Til We Free Us: Abolitionist Organizing and Transforming Justice, by Mariame Kaba, 2021. This book is a collection of writings and interviews encouraging us to consider our ideas around justice, and how we can organize our communities to abolish carceral industrial systems. Sage quotes Mariame Kaba in their interview – 'Hope is a discipline'.

Defund the Police, Invest in Community Care – A Guide to Alternative Mental Health Responses, by Mimi Kim, Megyung Chung, Shira Hassan, and Andrea J. Ritchie, 2021. A report, referenced by Sage, that explores anti-carceral mental health tools and interventions. www.interruptingcriminalization.com/non-police-crisis-response-guide

The Fireweed Collective. Sage mentioned the Fireweed Collective as an example of a self-sufficient community mental health initiative. They offer mental health education and mutual aid that prioritizes people of colour and healing justice. https://fireweedcollective.org

CAT-911. Another collective noted by Sage as an example of community-led, anti-carceral, transformative peace building. CAT-911 – which stands for Community Action Teams – operates in Southern California. https://cat-911.org

Ericka Hart. Sage quotes Hart in our discussion – 'Your queerness does not absolve your racism.' They are a queer, polyamorous, non-binary femme, who is also a writer, educator, model, and activist. They can be found on social media @IhartEricka and on their podcast *Hoodrat to Headwrap: A Decolonized Podcast.*

Black Identities and White Therapies: Race, Respect and Diversity, edited by Divine Charura and Colin Lago, 2021. This collection of critical essays draws attention to the colonial history and present of therapy with calls for new models of training future practitioners. It's an essential read for all therapists in training and practice.

Supporting Trans People of Colour: How to Make Your Practice Inclusive, by Sabah Choudrey, 2022. This book offers an accessible and comprehensive overview of how therapists and other professionals can create the safest spaces possible for trans people of colour, and keep intersectionality at the centre of their work. I keep it on my desk in my therapy office at all times.

Support for Trans Youth with Emily Waldron

An introduction to Emily

Emily (she/her) is a young trans woman living in England. She has been a staunch advocate for trans youth since she was 9 years old, working closely with organizations such as Mermaids and Amnesty International. When she's not advocating for trans rights she plays on several football teams – although, sadly, with the UK Supreme Court ruling in 2025 regarding single-sex spaces, Emily has now been banned from playing in one of her teams, to the shock and sadness of all of her teammates. She also creates trans-themed crafts, recently winning LGBTQ+ Young Business Person of the Year at the Gaydio Pride Awards 2024.

I first heard of Emily's activism several years ago, when she was forced to leave school due to transphobic bullying. Sadly, Emily's experience is not uncommon. Transphobic bullying in education is both extremely common (Witcomb *et al.*, 2019; De Pedro, Shim-Pelayo, and Bishop, 2019) and extremely detrimental to long-term mental health (Formby, 2013), and it often comes from both peers and teachers alike (Reynolds, 2022). Transphobic violence in schools is a growing concern (Gallardo-Nieto *et al.*, 2021) at the same time as rights are being stripped from young trans people across the UK

(Parsons, 2020; Thomas, 2024; Ferreira, 2024). This is especially true in the wake of the Cass Review, an NHS-commissioned review that led to a ban on privately prescribed puberty blockers for trans and gender questioning children in the UK (Madrigal-Borloz, 2023; Horton, 2024), as well as the closure of the Tavistock Gender Identity Clinic, the only NHS service that offered gender-affirming care to patients under 17 years of age (Pritilata, 2022).

Since leaving school Emily has spoken loudly and proudly on the impact of transphobic bullying and the positive impact of trans people in sports. I've admired Emily's activism and braveness over social media and knew she would have interesting things to say about trans rights in sport, education, and mental health.

Emily's mum, Emma, also joined us for the interview to provide some moral support and back-up information. Emma was just as lovely as Emily, and it seems like the support she provides her daughter is invaluable.

Emily's interview

Emily: I'm Emily and I'm 15. I enjoy doing stuff that's good for my mental health, and stuff that keeps me outdoors, like exercise. I like to get out and about, and I enjoy spending time with my pets – I absolutely adore them. I love to do advocacy work; that's one of the things that brings me a lot of joy. I like to play a lot of games, as well.

Katy: What kind of games do you like to play?

Emily: I like to play *FIFA*. I like *Rainbow Six Siege*, which is a shooter game. I don't mind a bit of *Minecraft* because that's really relaxing.

Katy: Yeah, that's pretty chill!
I first became aware of you and your story when you were forced

to leave school due to bullying. Do you want to tell me what that experience was like for you?

Emily: It was sad, it really was. It was hard to get by. It was hard to study. It was even hard to do things I enjoy. It was like I was in jail; I was just kind of locked up in my room, sat in bed all day. It was tough times. We had to find any little thing that brought me out of my room, at first, just doing anything to keep me distracted and entertained while we waited to see where we were gonna go with everything. Eventually, that led to doing things that would get me outside, even if it was just going to a museum or out for lunch. It was all the little things that made me feel a bit more human. I tried to do anything that made me feel good – we tried to do as much as possible.

It was quite a difficult time for everyone, because it meant doing a lot of new things, like homeschooling with my mum. That must have been difficult for her to get started, because it was very difficult for me, too. It meant having to stay home more often. It took up a lot of our time. It was a bit of a difficult start, but it's obviously gotten much easier now, and everything worked out in the end. But it was still a really difficult time to get through.

Katy: I can imagine. It sounds like it was a horrible time, but it also sounds like your family has been a really good support network.

Emily: My mum, my dad, and my brother, they've all helped me as much as they can. There's also my nan, and then I've got an older brother and his girlfriend. They've always been there around us to help, for as long as they have been able to. Since I first met all the people in my family, they've all been there for me and supported me and loved me unconditionally.

Katy: I'm so glad! That sounds like it's been so important.

Emily: It would have been much more difficult without them.

Katy: What other kinds of support do you have in your life right now?

Emily: I've got my group of friends around where I live. I've also got some friends who I went to secondary school with who I still speak to, because they wanted me to stay but they knew that I couldn't, so we made sure to keep in touch. Every now and again we'll meet up and see each other. It's the same with some of my friends from primary school, the way I still speak to them. They've always supported me, and their parents have always been supportive of me. They've always just understood me – they've always had good attitudes towards me, and I appreciate them.

There's also the football team I play for, TRUK United. They've helped me get through a lot of tough times. Whenever I've been down in the dumps, and we've been down for the game, it's been such a mood lifter. It's nice being around the transgender community, and anyone in the LGBTQ+ community, and any allies in general. They're always lovely to have around.

Katy: Speaking of football, what is it like to be a trans person in sport right now?

Emily: With everything that's going on – with people trying to have us banned – it's really, really frustrating. It makes my blood boil. It's like trying to take away joy; it's like taking sweets off a baby. It's taking the important stuff from the vulnerable, letting people have fewer things that help them. If I didn't have football during the time I was out of school, I think I'd probably have stayed as sad as I was at the start, or not too far off it. Sports was one of the main things that was keeping me happy outdoors, and even indoors. It was everything to do with football, whether it's playing FIFA online, training in the house, playing outdoors, or the matches with TRUK – it's always been there for me.

Being a trans person in sport, I think it's really important to keep playing and keep trying to fight for the right to be able to keep playing. It's the most important thing to be doing right now.

Katy: Sport is such an important thing to so many people, maybe especially to vulnerable people, to oppressed people. It's important to be able to express yourself in that way, to be able to play, to be able to compete, all of it. What is it that you like about football?

Emily: The first time I remember seeing it on TV I got lost into the game, and I ended up wanting to play it, and then I was playing it all the time, and it took a little chunk of my heart and sat in it. Having a football team, watching the games, it can be really fun! Other than, you know, some of the bad outcomes of the results in games, that can be a bit frustrating!

Katy: [Katy laughs] For sure! Aside from TRUK, who do you support?

Emily: I'm a big Liverpool fan. We've recently had two big losses, so that's been a bit annoying.

Katy: No, I get that. This is a Tottenham Hotspur household. [Both grimace and laugh]

When things get you down, what makes you feel resilient? What makes you feel empowered in the face of anti-trans oppression?

Emily: Advocacy. I think it could possibly be my favourite thing to do, in all honesty. Trans advocacy is really important at the minute with everything that's going on. Whether it's health care, sports, or just generally human rights, I think it's really important to have it fought for.

I think it's for that reason that I know I've got to fight further. Discrimination makes me want it all more, because I'm very competitive. It makes me want to fight stronger and harder to be able to have the same equal rights as any human being.

Katy: You're really making a difference. Do you want to tell me more about your advocacy work?

Emily: I think the first thing I worked on was *If I Had a Voice* (a crowdfunder campaign organized by Mermaids, featuring a video of Emily talking about her experiences of transphobic media when she was 11 years old)?

Emma (Emily's mum): No, I think it was *Butterfly* (the 2018 ITV drama series about a young trans girl, which was inspired by the charity work done by Mermaids).

Emily: Oh, *Butterfly*! The Mermaids mental health TV show. That was ages ago!

Emma: You were 9!

Emily: That was six years ago! That's a while back. I've always felt that it was just something I had to do, so, when I had that first chance to do some advocacy for the show *Butterfly*, it just felt right. It felt great seeing that, and seeing what Mermaids were doing with it.

It was a three-part drama. I remember watching all the episodes the moment they came out. It held a very big part of my heart, and I can't really let that bit go. I know it's always going to stick there with me, same as any work that I've done within mental health.

I think advocacy around mental health has been really important. I like thinking of what makes people happy and, in general, what people can do to support other people and to boost people's mental health. It's extremely important to work within that area, and the whole health care situation. With how things are going, that's going to have a huge negative impact on a lot of good people. I think that's quite devastating, with everything that's happening, and what's happened already within the community's health care for young trans people. Not only that – now there's the Cass Review. That's a big deal at the minute. I've really, really hated seeing everything happen with that – it's been quite upsetting. Things like this are the reason it is really important to keep working in advocacy. It's really important that people get to have their rights.

I've always known I was meant to be born how I am, to be a girl. That's always stuck with me, and it's always felt right, and it's always been in my head. It's who I want to be. It's who I am. I am this. I've known for a very long time, and it's really horrible to see rights and health care and stuff like that just slowly get taken away, just because of who I am.

Katy: I think the kind of advocacy you do is so important. It's always been needed, and I think that now it's going to be needed more than ever, especially with stuff like the Cass Review.

Emily: It's devastating.

Katy: I know it's made a lot of people very worried, including me.

Emily: Let's just hope that everything can go the right way.

Katy: I hope so, too. We have a lot of good people fighting, including you. While things are especially difficult right now, what does self-care look like for you?

Emily: What do I do with self-care? I think one of the most important things I like to do is have a bath bomb. Having a nice, hot bubble bath, it really relaxes me. And face and skincare – that plays a big part, especially when I'm relaxing with a bit of spa music. Every now and again I try on different bits of makeup – I thinks it's always fun to try new things.

Playing games, as well – for me that relieves a lot of stress. I've got a lot of stress toys as well, because that helps quite a lot. I enjoy little bits of puzzle solving, because it takes up a lot of time, it's distracting from the stress, and I enjoy doing it quite a lot.

What else? Oh, yeah, arts and crafts! Obviously, I love that. I enjoy doing that because whenever I feel down, I get to make a lot of new things and try stuff with my mum. That's really important for my self-care, spending time with my family, because they've helped me out from the beginning, and it's important that family sticks together. That's a very big, huge part of my life – my family and friends and everything I've made along the way. You've got to try and hold on to that, and make sure you know what your wins are, and what's important to you, and to have the right priorities of what keeps you safe and happy with your mental health. So, for me, family and friends play a huge part of that.

It also helps to have a lot of playtime with the family pets. I think they enjoy it, as well, because I think they can also have their low times. I always think it must be tough for the animals as well, because they don't have a voice. I always used to think about it as a kid – what would animals do for fun? I relax while playing with them and being there for them, because I absolutely love them, and hopefully they feel the same way about me.

Katy: I'm sure they do. Your ferret's famous now in the House of Commons, right?

Emma: The Ferret Filibuster! (This was a 2024 filibuster in which

Labour MPs blocked an anti-trans bill by discussing the best names for pet ferrets. Emily's pet ferret got a shout-out.)

Emily: [Emily laughs] Oh, that was fun! We've started crafting stuff about the ferrets now; we've made T-shirts and everything! Anything we can put a ferret on, we have!

Emma: She's a wonderful pet.

Emily: She's absolutely lovely. She can get in the way, and she can be quite funny, but we love her for it. Although she does spend a lot of time trying to escape the house. She's been successful a few times, but we always get her back. She just runs through people's back gardens and ends up about a two-minute walk away. It's always quite funny when we find her, but she does have us stressed out quite a lot when it happens. We love her a lot.

Katy: So cute!
    Is there anything that you would like to say to other young trans people?

Emily: I think it's super-important that young trans people try and stay on top of their mental health, and prioritize their self-care as much as possible.
    It's also important to find the right people to support you. Whether you're going through tough times, or anything isn't feeling right, or you're struggling, it's extremely important to try and have people around you. If family or friends aren't an option for you, it's about trying to find a community. It's trying to find support groups or places where you can go to meet people within the trans community, or just any allies in general.

Katy: I really like the idea that you can find self-care in community care, and vice versa. I think that's really important to remember.

How would you like the adults and the systems around you to be fighting for change?

Emily: Oh, that's a good one! [Katy laughs] I think supporting good charity work is really important, and having that around. But mostly I think it's really important to see us – to listen to trans kids – because it's our future that they're talking about. Many charities are not talking to us about it – they're talking to other people about it, and that's really frustrating. I remember we got asked to speak about that, didn't we?

Emma: Yeah, and then you went and they said there'd been a mistake, that it was a mix-up.

Emily: They said that I wouldn't be able to be spoken to. That really frustrated the both of us quite a lot, and it upsets me, because I was getting quite excited to finally be able to have the chance to speak out, to tell people what young trans people need and the support that we could have. The fact that they just threw me out, they kicked me to the curb, and just decided to say, 'No, you can't be here'. Those people spoke *for* me, instead of speaking *to* me, and that's really upsetting.

Katy: That's horrible. I'm sorry.

Emily: I think it's also important to have trans support groups come out and say what they've heard from us, and to use what they've got around them to help others.

It's important to inform others because people that know nothing about trans people keep talking about us. That annoys me. It's always people who know nothing about the trans community, or don't even know what the word really means, that are the worst. They talk about the trans community and act like they know what's best when it doesn't affect them. They talk about the most irrelevant stuff, like what clothes we wear, instead of something important. They have no idea what they're talking about, and that frustrates me so much. I think that people within the trans community, and allies, should be the ones to speak out about young trans people – non-binary people, as well. It's really, really important that the community can come together and be allowed to speak out. It's just very frustrating that people try to deflect us. That's the way they try their best to work around us. This is our lives that they're talking about! And it's speaking for us, instead of speaking to us, that creates this awful propaganda. That gets on my nerves.

Katy: Understandably so. There's so much purposeful misinformation out there from people who have no idea what they're talking about.

Emily: Yeah, there's a million of them. It's been great to have a voice here.

Katy: Thank you so much for taking the time to do this with me.

Emily: Thank you for listening. I've enjoyed this.

Katy's post-interview thoughts

Chatting to Emily about her systems of support was a delight, and I especially enjoyed hearing about how Emily has coped with her experiences of transphobia through exercise and sports. Participation in sports is another important area of life that trans people are increasingly demonized in and excluded from (Chan *et al.*, 2024), with no solid evidence base that this exclusion increases fairness for anyone (Jones *et al.*, 2016b). Sports are often excellent for mental health and community care, both in general and for young trans people in particular (DeChants *et al.*, 2024), so Emily's experiences with teams like TRUK United FC are important for the whole community. Everyone deserves to play, whether they're amazing or less than athletic like me (Lees, 2019), so it's wonderful to see Emily continuing to play well and have fun. I'm looking forward to seeing more of her wins in the future.

If you'd like to know more

@emz_crafts_ on Instagram. Emily's arts and crafts shop, where she raises money to fund her trans advocacy and travel to TRUK matches.

TRUK *United FC*. TRUK are an all-inclusive football team spearheaded by Trans Radio UK, with the aim of bringing the trans community together to play. https://trukunitedfc.com

If I Had a Voice, by Mermaids. This was a project aiming to boost the voices of trans youth and combat sensationalist misinformation about trans and children in the UK media. Emily's video was a central part of the campaign, 'Give transgender children like Emily a voice #IfIHadAVoice'. https://youtu.be/xhAkcoSQP34?si=-PgZIEwV5oi9pA5A

Ferret Filibuster. Emily mentions her pet ferret's role in the iconic Ferret Filibuster, in which transphobic bills were blocked from being heard by several members of the UK parliament who filibustered by talking at length about their pets. It was a heart-warming display of allyship, and you can read more about the event in this article by the fantastic Erin Reed from *Erin in the Morning*. www.erininthemorning.com/p/private-gender-affirming-care-ban

Autistic Queer Liberation with Gem Kennedy

An introduction to Gem

Gem (they/them) is genderqueer, neuroqueer, AuDHD, and witchy, which are all interlocking aspects of their transformational well-being work. They have many strings to their bow, including one-to-one coaching, home-education facilitation, Emotional Freedom Technique certification, podcasting, and advocacy work, all of which channel their passion for personal growth, community care, and social change. They prioritize accessibility in their life's work, not just for others but for themself, ensuring there's 'nothing about us without us' in their work and helping their clients and community to live in alignment with the truest expression of themselves.

Gem's pull to work with autistic queer clients is not surprising, seeing as there are so many of us looking for support (Dewinter *et al.*, 2017). Even while so many autistic people are LGBTQ+ (Holmes *et al.*, 2022; Weir, Allison, and Baron-Cohen, 2021), it's still difficult to access appropriate care that speaks to the wholeness of that experience (Cooper *et al.*, 2023). It's also no surprise that so many queer autistic people are seeking help to feel more connected with our emotions and our bodies; the stigma of both queerness and neurodivergence (Wallisch *et al.*, 2023; George and Stokes, 2018), the social and sensory stressors of self-understanding and queer self-expression (Lewis *et al.*, 2021), and high levels of masking and hiding oppressed identities (Hillier *et al.*, 2019) can disconnect us from how our bodies feel and exist in a world not built for us (Grove *et al.*, 2023). Even though these are very common experiences for queer people, they are also frequently derided (Holmes *et al.*, 2022; Khudiakova and Chasteen, 2022), and queer autistic people often find themselves being denied appropriate care (Jones, Hamilton, and Kargas, 2024; Bruce, Munday, and Kapp, 2023; Fortunato *et al.*, 2022). Neurodivergent queer mental health practitioners, too, can find it difficult to find accessible training and work, while neurotypical 'experts' on autism are centred (Walker, 2021).

All this gives Gem's inclusive, authentic, consent-based work a little extra magic. I've been lucky enough to receive some of that magic myself as a client, and I can say for certain that the work we've done together has been transformative for me. Because Gem has worked as my coach, and I their coachee, there was some hesitation before I asked them to be a part of this project. I knew they would be wonderful to interview, and I was excited to share their important insights, but I took some time to think about how this might affect our therapeutic relationship. This was something we pondered together before Gem officially joined this project, and we were able to bring a sense of mutual enthusiasm and care to the interview.

Gem's interview

Gem: I'm Gem! I'm a transformational coach and also a facilitator. I'm not really sure how I would define the spiritual part of some of the stuff that I do at the moment – I'm still figuring it out – but I'm witchy, and that's an increasing part of my work. I'm genderqueer, trans, and non-binary. I'm 37. I live in Essex (England, UK).

I have two children. I'm a single parent. My children are home educated, so they've never been to school. They are 12 and 8. I don't really ever talk about them in my work – I'm always happy to talk about things in relation to them, but now they're always like, 'Why don't you ever talk about us?' [Both laugh] They're wanting me to talk more about them, but I am conscious of keeping them private.

I'm obviously neurodivergent, and I'm in a neurodivergent family. It's been maybe over the last six or seven years that we've been figuring that out. We started thinking about neurodivergence for specific family members, then more people have realized, so there's been lots going on in that time!

Katy: How would you describe your current work?

Gem: I would say that very different parts make up my work, but it feels like there's a cohesive aim.

As a coach, I work one-to-one with clients, and they tend to almost all be autistic and queer. That work obviously looks different depending on who I'm working with, but the strands are related to being queer, being autistic, and possibly other neurodivergences as well. There's often a witchy angle to some of the work that I'm doing with people, plus EFT (Emotional Freedom Technique, otherwise known as 'tapping'), as well as much more practical thinking about what they do at work, or how they make their lives more neurodivergent-friendly, depending on what people want. I also run post-diagnosis sessions for late-identified autistic adults.

I run courses and socials too for autistic adults through an organization called Thriving Autistic.

The last part of my work is that, two days a week, I work as a facilitator in a self-directed setting for home-educated young people. In one of the settings I'm a co-lead, and that's with ages 5 to 11-ish. The other setting is for ages 10 to 16 – that setting is newer, and I'm a facilitator at that one.

Katy: That's so much important work!

Gem: Hopefully, yeah! [Both laugh]

Katy: To start with your coaching work – what brought you to trans-formational coaching, EFT, and the one-to-one strand of your work?

Gem: In 2016 or 2017 – quite some time ago – I had a friend through the home-ed network who had been training to be a transforma-tional coach, and she was looking for people to do sessions with. I was at this point in my life where I was figuring out a lot of stuff and was like, 'I'd like to do that!' We had about six sessions together and during that time I found it so helpful. I was at a point in my life where I had quite young children, and I hadn't really had much of a chance to figure it all out. Life was very intense, and my children were really little, so coaching sessions were a nice space to figure out what was going on with me and what I wanted to do, or not do.

In the last session I remember feeling like she'd helped me with lots of things, and I was feeling like I was in a really good position with stuff, but there was one thing that I had never really talked to anyone about, and I didn't know if she'd help me. It was around body-related stuff and eating disorder stuff. I did bring it up, and talking to her about that changed so much. Looking back, I'm so surprised that it felt so new to me, but the fact that she listened and reassured me that other people experienced that too, I was shocked.

From there, I experienced what I now know to be hyperfocus. I was finding out everything I could related to the anti-diet movement, so I was reading things like Megan Jayne Crabbe's *Body Positive Power* and thinking, 'Oh my god, this is all so good!' I went into a really deep dive around it. I fell in love with the work of Charlotte Cooper and lots of other people who talk about fat activism. I kept thinking that I'd love to do this work with other people, because there's so many people that are affected by diet culture, and helping people with that would be so cool. I decided to train as a coach, and I started doing that work, and it's all grown from there.

When I was thinking about body liberation, I was also wondering, what about queer people who experience these problems? Where are they having these conversations? What are they saying? Those questions led me to making a zine, and then that turned into a podcast, which is called *Queers and Co.*

Then I learned more about my own neurodivergence, and that learning showed up in my work, too. So, it's all snowballed!

Katy: It sounds like this side of your work has really grown with all of the discoveries that you've made for yourself.

Gem: Definitely! It felt like so many things folded in along the way. Then spirituality came into it, which included figuring out how you connect with your sense of self instead of just doing things 'properly'.

I don't know that I would have been able to do any of that if I hadn't already been in the home-ed community, and learning about consent and self-direction, and how important that was for children, and then also applying it to myself. It was good to realize that I haven't finished learning, that I could learn and do things that follow my interests.

Now, looking back, it seems like a really natural progression, but at the time I had no idea where it would end up.

Katy: I can definitely see the connecting thread around autonomy, and congruence, and being at home in yourself.

Gem: Definitely!

Katy: Would you like to tell me more about how you become involved in queer body liberation activism?

Gem: Around the time I was training to be a transformational coach, I was processing the end of my marriage. In the run up to all of that, I also had things around gender and sexuality coming up. I'd come out as bi when I was in my teens and then I hadn't done anything with that realization – it felt like it wasn't really an accessible part of my identity, for various reasons. As I learned more about how I'd kept myself contained because of diet culture, other things started to pop up, and I realized there was so much I hadn't explored for myself. I'd remember how I used to feel when identified as bi. It all started coming out, and coming together. I think the coming together of those two things was helped by really hearing other people talk about more radical politics around bodies and queerness, and what that connection means.

Katy: It's so interesting how making space for yourself in one area can open up so much more. What was your journey towards understanding yourself as a neurodivergent queer person?

Gem: I'd say the queerness came first, for sure. I was already identifying as queer, and then as non-binary, and then later as genderqueer/trans. The neurodivergent realizations came later.

When my eldest was about 5 years old, she had a really bad autistic burnout and, at that time, I had no idea what was going on. I was like, 'We can't leave the house – what is happening?!' All the doctor said was to take her to a counsellor. They wouldn't even come to the house to see her when I couldn't get her out of the house. This was happening in the middle of all the other stuff, too. I was like, 'Okay, this can't continue. I need to know what is happening.' I did another hyperfocus to figure out all the things, and worked out that what was going on for her was sensory processing related, and that she's autistic. SPD (sensory processing disorder) isn't a recognized condition in the UK or in the US *Diagnostic and Statistical Manual of Mental Disorders* (DSM), so I found someone who was an occupational therapist who specialized in sensory processing in the Midlands (UK), and we went there. It was very difficult to get my daughter there because she was in so much burnout, but she went and had this assessment and, from there, everything started to fall into place. The specialists agreed that, with her sensory burnout, it was highly likely that she's also autistic, so she was diagnosed as autistic.

At that time I had a conversation with Kieran Rose, who is also known as 'The Autistic Advocate'. We were talking about it all and he was saying, 'You know, it's really common that at least one parent is also autistic...' And I was like, [in a tone of bright naivety] 'Oh, that's so interesting!' [Both laugh] And then I was like, 'Is it me? I don't know. I'm not sure if it's me.' It took me a lot longer to work out how neurodivergence shows up in other people who are not white cis men. It took a while of really seeing and realizing that a lot of what I could see in my daughter was also my experience as a young person.

School refusal is a good example of a classically observed autistic trait. Because my daughter hadn't gone to school there was no school refusal. I hadn't thought of myself as being a school refuser, either, but now I remember literally begging my mum not to send me to school. My mum didn't know what else to do, because there wasn't any support in those days – or, at least, the support wasn't quite the same. I hated school, but I was reading when I was 2 years old and having really intense conversations when I was 18 months old, and that was always just a bit of a family joke, just an anecdote. Looking back, all these pieces started slotting into place, and I was like, 'Oh my god, I was so autistic!' [Both laugh]

Katy: I'm laughing because that's really relatable!

Gem: Right! And seeing all those things together, rather than just judging myself because I was someone who didn't stop talking from a really young age, or whatever – it started to make so much sense.

So that was the autism part. There were still parts of my experience that weren't explained by autism entirely. That's where I started to explore other aspects of myself and my childhood – you know, I was always described as a daydreamer, or being a bit spacey, as a kid. I struggled with remembering things. I still leave my stuff and walk off and forget things. There's a lot of attention deficit hyperactivity disorder (ADHD) stuff that made sense.

Katy: What was your journey like as you realized you're genderqueer and trans?

Gem: I came out as non-binary in 2019. It came about when I tried to apply for a trademark for *Queers and Co.* I'm now so aware of the complex stuff around trademarking that I'm not sure I would bother to do it now because of all the ways it's not ideal, but I didn't know any better at the time. The application got turned down, and their reason was because the word 'queer' was offensive to modern British values. I remember being like, 'Fuck you! [Both laugh] What are you even talking about?' My feeling, at that point, was that 'queer' is a great label that I felt really connected to, and I knew lots of other people did, too. So, I started a petition, and that got picked up by change.org as one they promoted. From there, it ended up being in some papers.

The reason I'm telling you this is because that was the first time that I was like, 'Oh, something doesn't feel good.' I was seeing myself on websites like thepinknews.com, where the headline was something like, 'Woman campaigns for queer trademark change'. I felt so gross. I was like, 'Oh, no, that's not me. Who are they talking about?'

It made me realize that I've had these periods in my life where I've been deeply averse to wearing skirts, for example, and I've had other times where I will only wear skirts and wouldn't even dream of wearing trousers. I always put that down to having a bad relationship with my body, and all those awful 1990s fashion tips about 'looking thin' and all that shit.

Katy: All that 'never wear stripes' bullshit?

Gem: Exactly. Like 'black is slimming', and all that rubbish. But then, actually, I realized that I was not experiencing gender in the same way as others. I had all of this internalized stuff around it. I remembered having my hair cut short when I was maybe 12, and wanting to like it, but also not feeling feminine enough for other people, and knowing other people would judge me about that. So many memories came back to me!

From 2019 I started using she/they pronouns and then I switched to just using they/them. It feels so much better.

Now, what's been interesting is noticing that my gender fluctuates day to day, so I don't always feel the same way. Not that I assume everyone's gender feels the same all the time, but I noticed that it changes for me. I'm in a period now where I feel much more aligned with how I present on the outside.

It's also been interesting to discover I find genderqueerness really attractive in other people. That's probably because I've done some work to undo a lot of the really problematic things we're told about gender and attraction.

What's been particularly interesting is that I was in a relationship where I didn't feel affirmed in my gender for a few months. Everything else was really good. That experience opened up something in me where I then had this massive swing away from my usual feeling of alignment, where I had so much really difficult gender stuff coming up. I was considering things that I had always thought I didn't really want for myself – like I should definitely start taking testosterone, or I should definitely have top surgery. I still don't know where I'm at with those things. I have no judgement on whether they're good or bad – they're just gender-affirming health care – but I didn't think that I needed them for myself. I thought I'd got to a fixed point in my fluidity, weirdly, where I understood it. Having that massive kind of swing where figuring out my transness started to feel really difficult was scary. I had a lot of gender dysphoria. I feel like, now, I've come back to a more balanced place of being able and interested to learn more about my gender, but not feeling like I urgently need the things that I thought I did a few months ago. It's been a real lesson, for me, that even when you think you've got it figured out, you might not have. I think, in a way, maybe I was a bit cocky about it – like, 'Yeah, I'm just genderfluid! I know where I'm at with this!' And then I totally didn't!

Katy: It sounds like not being fully affirmed really affected how you were able to affirm yourself.

Gem: I think so too. Maybe that's why things I hadn't considered before suddenly felt like a way to really show who I was? It's like I was trying to find something extra-affirming.

I also find it so interesting that this other person did not intend to make me feel like this. They are a brilliant person. How well people deal with others' gender can depend so much on where they are with their own stuff, and how far they've figured out gender for themselves. We all have internalized transphobia that we need to pay attention to. But, yeah, that feeling of not being affirmed was really intense and not good. It took me a while to figure out, probably also because I'm an autistic person. It took me a while to figure out why something didn't feel quite right.

Things feel a lot more 'right' again. Next week I'm starting an online act development course with Rubyyy Jones. Rubyyy is this really cool performer and teacher who teaches all kinds of cool stuff, like emceeing and drag makeup. This online course is about act development and I'm basically leaning totally into my drag king era. It feels like a really good place to be. I started doing drag makeup after that relationship ended as a way to connect with my masculinity. Having a connection with that experience really helped – when I put the makeup on, I don't want to take it off. I feel like doing drag is going to be a really helpful way to play with what it means to lean into different parts of my gender identity and, hopefully, we can figure out a bit more.

Katy: That's so cool! Do you know what kind of act you might want to do? I recently saw a video of a drag king doing an act as a naughty Freud.

Gem: Oh, cool! That's interesting – very highbrow! [Both laugh]

I had two different ideas from very different places. One of them I don't think I'm going to do, but I'm going to pocket it for later, maybe – that was around being the queer dad that a lot of people didn't have. I don't have a relationship with my dad – so, what would it be like to have a dad who was really affirming and really supportive? Lots of queers are in the Shit Dad Club, so I think that would be a nice act. But then, talking about it with friends, they're like, 'Why would you bring your dad into it? Why not do something that is really about you, and about how you connect with yourself?' And I was like, 'Oh, my god, that makes so much sense!' I want to prioritize this creative opportunity and make it about something new.

So now, the act I want to develop is gonna be more at the intersections of weightlifting/gym bro/hot genderqueer vibes. It's going to be more sexy. The 'queer dad' act would be a nice thing to do, and I think that is a lot of where I sit in terms of wanting to be supportive and kind, but actually the idea of playing with a character that is an alter ego, something different for me, feels quite good.

Katy: It sounds like you're excited to learn in this group!

I know that a lot of your own group work and facilitation is about finding the joy and the magic in being neurodivergent. What brings you and your clients queer joy?

Gem: There's a few things. I think what's really bringing me joy at the moment is allowing myself to be enthusiastic. I think I am an enthusiastic person anyway but, sometimes, and especially in the past, I have put a lid on that enthusiasm and tried to seem more level, or not as excited about things. Right now I'm really enjoying things like...I sometimes see stoats or weasels – I'm never sure which is which – running around outside, and it just makes me so happy, because they're so cute that I want to just squish them! Obviously I wouldn't, and they'd probably bite me! [Both laugh] But things like animals, or fidgets, or things that feel really nice or look really nice. I'm really enjoying just allowing myself to enjoy those things.

In the last six months or so I've been figuring out more around sensory stuff for myself. For me, weightlifting brings me so much joy because it's so much intense pressure on my body. It's almost like having a massage or something. I feel so regulated afterwards. That's made me really happy, to know that I can actually just lift really heavy things and it makes my body feel calm. Not even in a mental health way, although it contributes to that, but more in a very regulated sensory way.

Katy: That totally makes sense to me. I have a friend who is a strongwoman with ADHD, and she says that weightlifting is a great way to stim!

Gem: Exactly. I've heard that ADHD people are often better at weightlifting. They can lift heavier than neurotypical, non-ADHD people can, which I am really interested in.

It's also just so fun! It always makes me think of all that body shame and exercise trauma from PE at school, and struggling so much but masking and trying to pretend that I can do those things while finding it really difficult… Exercise has been really complicated for me and it's so nice now to connect with it in a different way. I just want to lift heavy shit because it makes me feel regulated, rather than all that other stuff that is often supposed to come with exercise. I'm really enjoying that.

Another thing that brings me joy right now? Jelly. I really love jelly. I don't like eating it, I just like looking at it. It's so good when it wobbles! Oh my god! I love exploring sensory stuff and stim toys with my clients.

Another thing that I'm realizing the importance of, and that I've maybe taken for granted in recent years, is having other neurodivergent or queer people in your life. I think I'm so lucky, because of the work that I do, that I'm just constantly surrounded by queer autistic people. Whereas, speaking to some people when I'm running a social or speaking to one-to-one clients, I know others who don't have anyone who's queer or autistic in their lives. I'm really just realizing the importance of that. It sounds so silly to say that – I think I knew it for myself, then found my community, and then was like, 'Everyone has this!' But, obviously, they don't. I'm thinking about how I can be more involved with helping that to happen for everyone. How do we find people who we can connect with as queer, trans, neurodivergent people? Obviously, I would like to be everyone's friend, but that's probably not the most helpful thing! [Both laugh] My point is that shared community brings queer neurodivergent people a lot of joy. Feeling affirmed and understood – it's a basic human need, right?

Katy: For sure. I get the feeling that is also a lot of what's happening in your facilitation work, and in the unschooling work that you do as well. I imagine a big part of that work is about finding like-minded, like-brained community.

Gem: That aspect of it feels really important. I think community, and being able to live in alignment with yourself, are important sources of peace and joy. Whether it's right from the beginning – like not having to go to school, and feeling held but connected to your own sense of autonomy and agency – up to finding out much later in life that you're queer or autistic or neurodivergent.

This is probably because, for such a long time, I didn't feel connected to myself or a sense of community. I felt like an alien for as long as I could remember. Finding my community and feeling supported like that, it's just so important.

Katy: It's great that you have that community, and also that you can help other people to find theirs, too.

Gem: I really don't think I realized how important it was, either. It's almost like, not having had it growing up, I didn't think of it as necessary until I had it as an adult. I had friends, but I didn't have a sense of community. I didn't feel an intense sense of connection with a lot of the people around me. It wasn't until I was in a home-ed community that I actually started making proper friends that I really felt understood me. It's so sad that so many people don't have that. It's really rubbish.

Also, as a queer single parent, I've been realizing the importance of queerness in all this. The idea of the nuclear family in straight culture is that you've always got your people there for you, because you've got a husband, and you've got kids, and actually I don't have that. There's a lot of my family that I don't have contact with, and also now, as a single parent, I don't have a partner to rely on or to take the place of those kinds of connections. So I really have learned to prioritize and cherish my friendships and my connections with my chosen family members.

Katy: I'm so glad you and your kids have your home-ed community. What does your work in your home-ed community involve?

Gem: My home-ed work is about children's rights and the importance of self-direction. Finding out about children's rights activism, specifically, was a huge life shift for me. This learning happened before all of the other realizations.

I was always worried about my eldest going to school. When my youngest was about 6 months old, I found out in a local parents group that home-ed was a thing, totally by chance. I genuinely hadn't heard of it existing in the UK. There was a home-ed group that was running near us, so we went along, and it was amazing. I felt really connected to the people, and to their ideas around how children are oppressed.

They spoke about how, even if people don't experience any other marginalization as they grow up, even if they're all the things that society prioritizes, the one thing that all people have experienced is childhood oppression. You know, it's perfectly fine for people to say, 'I don't like children.' As the world progresses, it would not be okay to say that about neurodivergent people, or disabled people, or people of colour. It really hit me that, from such a tiny age, children are not advocated for; they're treated as property of the parents. That comes from patriarchy – that the dad is the 'king' of the family, and the children are the property, and the mum is the stand-in for the patriarch when the patriarch is out at work. I really didn't want that for my kids. I'd already seen how the school system had damaged me, and I had been a shell of myself there – I found it so difficult.

The thing that I really love about unschooling and self-directed education is that people are treated as people. The adults who are in that situation, whether they're parents or facilitators, are partners to the children. They help them advocate for themselves, or find out what they need to learn, or what they want to do. They're not there being this parental control, deciding that everyone needs to learn maths today.

I think my children are a great example of what self-directed learning can look like, in that they know themselves really well. They're able to say what they need. They're able to call me out – I don't think I really do this very often at all, but if ever there's any incidents where I'll be like, 'I'm telling you to do it because I said so', they'll be like, 'Hold on a second, we don't do things that way.' They're able to talk to adults like they're other humans, rather than feeling like there's a hierarchy, and they have friendships with people of all ages, and not just in their year group. There are so many advantages.

Katy: It seems like you have kids that really trust themselves because of the work that you've put into all this. It sounds like your kids are putting hard work into this, too, and all of your community.

Gem: Exactly. It's definitely not just me – my kids have got really brilliant adults in their lives, and really brilliant kids in their lives, who also learn about consent and self-direction, and are able to advocate for themselves. It's not easy. It's definitely not easy being autistic and trying to do that stuff, especially when autistic people have so often learned to people-please or do whatever we need to do to fit in and not feel like aliens.

Home-ed feels so 'everyday' to us. We've been home-eding since my daughter was 5, and she's now 12. I forget that other people don't do it or don't know what it is, and so sometimes we get asked when we're out and about, 'Oh, you're not at school today?' And I'm like, 'Oh shit, not everyone knows that you don't have to go to school!'

The other thing that I would add to that is that there's often this narrative that you can only home-ed if you're privileged or have a lot of money. On the one hand, I hear that and understand that, but at the same time, for people like us, it really isn't a choice. I have worked so hard to try and get into a position that means it's possible for us. I changed almost every aspect of my working life in order for that to happen. It was not easy to make it work, but I genuinely don't think my kids would cope in school and so, for us, it's not a choice. Often people want to do this with their kids but think you have to earn loads of money, but I'm not loaded and I'm a single parent. It's just really important to me, and I have been able to make it work. I know not everyone can.

Katy: This all really has me thinking about how often I have conversations with my clients, where they'll have what I've learned are really common signs of childhood trauma, and they'll say, 'But I didn't have a traumatic childhood.' I think maybe all kids do, to some degree, because so much of what adults do to kids would be considered abusive if we did it to adults, even stuff that is so common. I watch kids get gaslit all the time. It's the really common stuff, like a kid falls over and says they hurt themselves, and the adults are like, 'No, you didn't. Come on, you're fine. Walk it off. Stop crying.' You wouldn't do that to an adult. It really teaches kids not to trust themselves.

Gem: I agree with what you're saying there about how society treats kids. I think all of us who've been through the school system for sure have school trauma. I'm sure there are some people who do enjoy school, but I don't think you can be in such an oppressive environment where you don't have agency and not experience some trauma.

I remember when I first started working in an office, I put my hand up to go to the toilet, and they were like, 'What are you doing?' It's just so prevalent. It's become so normalized in the school system that you can't eat when you're hungry. You can't move your body when you need to. You have to focus on particular things, which is hard enough for kids, but especially for neurodivergent kids. That structure of being assigned a book and then you have to learn it without doing anything else at all – it can be impossible for neurodivergent people to do that healthily. If we have no interest in something, it's really hard to manufacture that, day-in day-out.

Katy: I know that, even when I was interested in what I was learning – like, if I was given a book to learn from and it was the kind of book I'd really enjoy – I would still be putting all my energy into looking like I was focusing on the book, making sure I was turning the pages at the same speed as everybody else in the class, trying to make sure I was sitting still in a posture that looked like I was learning. I did all of that while being full of fear and anxiety that I was going to do it all wrong, and that I would be in trouble. I had to look like I was coping, instead of actually doing what I needed to cope.

Gem: Totally! There's an added layer of fear and frustration for neurodivergent kids in school, for sure. There's just so much to think about and to manage – oh, it's just exhausting. You couldn't pay me to go back to those times in my life.

My kids know that if at any point they wanted to go to school, they totally could. We talk about how that's an option for them but, whenever we have the conversation about it, they're like, 'Absolutely not! Why would I want to go there? I have choice, and freedom, and friends that understand me.' Some people do choose to go from home-ed into school, and that's totally legit as well, for various reasons. They might want to do that for their exams, for example.

I think the main thing is having an adult that will advocate for you and support your choices, because often children's choices aren't taken seriously, or they don't even have any choices to make. They can't even choose their hobbies often – they're just sent to swimming club or whatever. I think it's really a big thing.

Katy: Is there anything you'd recommend for adults who have school trauma?

Gem: Give yourself permission to do some self-direction. Let yourself pay attention to what you want and need in the moment, and do it.

Because of the way we're taught to grow up in schools, a lot of adults don't have a connection with what they want or need, especially if you're neurodivergent. Our understanding of our physical needs is taken away, and then there's this constant pressure from a really young age to decide what you want to do for the rest of your life. Kids are forced to make those choices. Some people really know what they want to do, and they do that, and that's great! Lots of people don't, especially when they're kids.

The thing that I really have appreciated learning about self-direction is to actually listen to myself and be able to connect with myself in terms of consent. I've been hearing what my yeses and noes and maybes are around particular things. Being a self-employed person, that's so great, because when I'm interested in something I can follow that thread and do something around it.

A really big part of the work that I love to do is helping people to reconnect with that sense of what they actually want for themselves. What do you want to do? If we're working towards stuff that we think other people think we should do, then it's not going to work – how are we going to be enthusiastic about that? It is much easier to follow your own interests and follow what feels good to you. I think that's what a lot of adults have no connection with.

Katy: While you help to transform yourself and your clients in the world, how do you like to take care of yourself?

Gem: To take good care of myself, I've had to relearn a lot of basic things that I feel like, for example, the school system does not help you to have. I've had to relearn my relationship with food and movement, for example. Right now, I'm trying to keep my life as simple as possible, and really listen to myself.

For example, if I book a social thing, I'll have anxiety about it. So, if it's in two months' time, I'll worry about it for two months, and the payoff is like, I might have a good time, but I also might just come home feeling exhausted and having worried about it for two months. I look after myself by properly listening to myself and thinking, 'Do I actually want to spend my energy on that? Probably not. Okay, then no, thanks.'

Another thing that is really meaningful to me in terms of self-care has been having a regular magic practice. For almost four years now, almost every Thursday, me and a friend meet to do magic together. For us, that includes a combination of visualization and tarot cards. Sometimes we have magic weekends, either at home or away somewhere, and that has been more transformative than almost any other thing that I've done to take care of myself. It helps me to feel more connected to myself and to the world. It feels like I'm constantly learning more about myself and what it means to be alive. There's always so much more to learn, and that's a really good way to take care of myself, I think.

Katy: You've mentioned your magic practice a few times, as self-care and as something you're folding into your work. What does that tend to look like with your clients?

Gem: As I've learned more, or felt more connected to having a personal spirituality, I've started to bring that more into my work.

Spark (Gem's monthly magical meetup online, which is now a monthly email newsletter) has been a really good way to explore that. What I'm really enjoying is creating spaces that aren't just supportive and affirming, but also have a magical element to them. For me, that is what *Spark* is. It's great being able to reflect on what happened last month with like-minded people who are making social change. The connections that potentially come from that are really great. I always feel energized to do it, and energized by doing it. I don't ever feel drained or tired afterwards – I just want to do it again!

I feel excited for how that energy can develop more in terms of how it can integrate across all of my work. I've enjoyed doing tarot and oracle pulls for people lately – that's such a cool experience.

Katy: This all sounds amazing, but I'm kind of sadly thinking about the last tarot pulls we have done… [Katy laughs] If you remember, when I drew a card thinking about how I wanted this book to go, I drew The Tower (a card often associated with catastrophe and destruction). You interpreted that as me writing something that prioritizes the destruction of the systems of power that hurt queer minds, and not as the book being a disaster, which helped!

Gem: I think it's really interesting, isn't it? During particularly bad times, like when I was getting divorced, I got The Tower so many times. It almost became comforting – an acknowledgement that it was okay to feel shit because things kept being shit, rather than being told that everything's fine.

It helps me to remember it's not predicting the future, it's offering you themes or things to be aware of. How you interpret all of this is self-directed!

Katy's post-interview thoughts

I really enjoyed this interview, and I've particularly enjoyed Gem's thinking regarding consent as both community care and self-care. Consent is something I prioritize in all of my relationships, especially my therapeutic relationships, but how often do I really ask myself for consent before I do things? How often do I truly let my life be entirely self-directed, without masking or shame? Trusting in your own ability to determine your day-to-day life, and your future, can be really regulating, especially when it feels like we often have so little control of our bodies and our safety. I made sure I intentionally did some self-direction after this interview, checking in to see what my neuroqueer self wanted and needed. I hope you can do that for yourself, too.

If you'd like to know more

Queers and Co. podcast, by Gem Kennedy. This is Gem's podcast, where they chat to a variety of amazing LGBTQ+ change-makers about what's most important to them. www.gemkennedy.com/podcast

Spark. Spark is Gem's neuroqueer monthly guided resource for all things witchy, reflective, and creative. www.gemkennedy.com/work/spark

Body Positive Power: Because Life Is Already Happening and You Don't Need Flat Abs to Live It, by Megan Jayne Crabbe, 2017. Gem mentioned they enjoyed reading this book while searching for anti-diet resources. This book is an accessible and congruent look at how body acceptance can help us find peace and joy.

Fat Activism: A Radical Social Movement, by Charlotte Cooper, 2016. Another book that Gem said helped them connect with anti-diet ideas. The book is an in-depth exploration into the politics of fatness, the everyday lives of fat people, and how fat activism ties undeniably into queer justice and feminism.

Thriving Autistic. A global not-for-profit organization designed to support autistic people in a variety of ways with a focus on inclusion and empowerment. Gem runs courses and socials for autistic adults through this organization. www.thrivingautistic.org

Kieren Rose, aka The Autistic Advocate. In our interview Gem noted that a conversation with Kieren Rose was instrumental to them thinking of themself as autistic. https://theautisticadvocate.com

@rubyyyjones on Instagram. Gem's drag act development course was run by Rubyyy Jones, who describes themself as a creator, consultant, and curator.

@pip.dream on Instagram. Pip Dream is the 'Drag King, Dreamboat, and Pedlar of Highbrow Stupidity' who performed the Freud-themed act that I mentioned to Gem, which still lives in my mind rent free.

Fat and Queer: An Anthology of Queer and Trans Bodies and Lives, edited by Miguel M. Moreles, Bruce Owens Grimm, and Tiff Ferentini, 2021. A book recommendation from me that picks up on many of Gem's thoughts around fatness, queerness, gender, embodiment, and empowerment.

LGBTQ+ Eating Disorder Treatment with Jess Sprengle

An introduction to Jess

Jess Sprengle (she/they) is a queer, gender-expansive, ADHD, eating disorder therapist with lived experience of eating disorder recovery. They also describe themself as a cat person, an avid reader, and a meme curator. As well as being a therapist and an online meme master, Jess is also an advocate, educator, consultant, and podcast host. Their life's work is about ensuring LGBTQ+ and neurodivergent folks can access relational and authentic eating disorder treatment, via one-to-one therapy in Texas and New Jersey, plus online advocacy worldwide. You might know them as @thecrankytherapist on social media, where they share memes about mental health, eating disorder recovery, daily life, and a behind-the-scenes look at what it's like to be a therapist, which is mostly that we're all a bit weird.

With eating disorders being so prevalent among LGBTQ+ people (Parker and Harriger, 2020), and especially with trans and/or non-binary individuals (Jones *et al.*, 2016a), I knew that Jess would have knowledge that LGBTQ+ people would need. Research has shown that all kinds of LGBTQ+ people are more likely to experience eating disorders than allocishet people (Nagata, Ganson, and Austin,

2020). Bisexual people and young trans people experience particularly high rates of disordered eating (Santonicollo and Rollè, 2024; Meneguzzo *et al.*, 2024; Connolly *et al.*, 2016). Among young trans people in particular, it has been found that trans men, non-binary people who were assigned female at birth, and multiracial people of all genders are more likely to show signs of disordered eating (Trevor Project, 2022). Experiencing discrimination and rigid appearance ideals – experiences that are, unfortunately, very common among all LGBTQ+ people (Meyer, 2003; Hendricks and Testa, 2012) – can make the chances of experiencing disordered eating much higher (Santonicollo and Rollè, 2024; Gordon *et al.*, 2019).

Like Jess – like many of us – I'm a queer, gender-expansive person who has healed, and is still healing, from disordered eating, so Jess's words, both over time and in this interview, resound powerfully and bittersweetly in many areas of my life. Interestingly, Jess and I are also both neurodivergent therapists who started their therapy career surprisingly young, and who work relationally with clients who are often neurodivergent, queer, and trans. Jess was the first collaborator that I interviewed for this book, and I wonder if you can read some of my eager nervousness in what Jess and I created together. I reached out to them after following them on social media for years and admiring their work – not just their right-on therapeutic takes, but also their humour, their meme-collecting, their excellent photos of their cats, and their commitment to solidarity and inclusivity in their online spaces. When I DMed them to see if they would be interested in being interviewed for the book, I was intimidated – I felt like I wasn't cool enough to ask this therapeutic rock star if they wanted to be involved with my project. I needn't have listened to my own imposter syndrome, as I got a warm and excited reply full of enthusiasm for the project. It turns out Jess had read my first published book, *The Trans Guide to Mental Health and Well-Being*, which I found pleasing and mortifying by degrees. I'm glad that the enthusiasm to chat together about LGBTQ+ eating disorder treatment, and more, was mutual.

Jess's interview

Jess: My name is Jess Sprengle. My pronouns are she/they.

One of the most important things about me is I'm a therapist. I work with folks with eating disorders, and I work very often with folks who are queer and trans who have eating disorders, and/or who are neurodivergent and have eating disorders. I have this nice little niche with the most wonderful clients!

I feel very fortunate to do the work that I do. I can't imagine doing anything else at this point, even when I'm tired and don't want to do it, because it has given me a lot of really good meaning to my own experiences. That's surprising, because I hear the worst things people have ever experienced, but knowing that people have a space to come to and actually be honest helps, and to me that definitely restores my faith in the future of humanity.

I did also just start a podcast with a therapist friend who is wonderful, and it is called *I'm Triggered*. We talk about media, and mental health portrayals in media, and we talk about triggers, and go into what that looks like both personally and on a more general scale. That's been a labour of love and a really big project, so that has occupied a lot of space in my life recently. It's at the top of my mind. I just recorded an episode earlier today, so that's a lot of what I'm doing right now.

So, in a nutshell, I am a therapist, I'm a little podcast person now, but also, yeah, I'm just a person! And I'm trying to think what else I would say about me. I am very much a cat person. I'm thoroughly a cat person, I like to say.

Katy: I'm also a cat person. I'm sorry if you can hear my cats clawing at the door. Apparently they want to meet you! [Both laugh]

Jess: Awwww! Really and truly, I think the most flattering and lovely feeling is when a cat is nice to you. Cats are discerning so, if a cat likes you, you're in business. You're a good person.

Katy: I think you have to be a special kind of person for cats to really like you.

Jess: I agree. I'm biased, because I have two cats, but I have a special love for the little felines. They're very silly.

Katy: Agreed! So, what kind of counselling do you practice?

Jess: I typically do individual therapy – so, one-to-one. I do sometimes meet with families but not as frequently.

Because working with eating disorders is so nuanced and complex, there's not really a lot of specific ways that I work with clients. Any time I teach people about working with eating disorders, there's a lot of frustration that's like, 'Why can't you teach me specific skills to work with eating disorders?' There are certain behavioural interventions that are useful, but at the end of the day it's such an individual problem, despite symptoms looking similar, that we really don't have any gold standard interventions or treatments, at least in my opinion. Some people really, really disagree. There's evidence-based practices for anorexia like CBT (cognitive behavioural therapy) and FBT (family-based therapy). No shade to any of those people, but I just do not find that those are approaches that really get to the heart of the problem.

I'm definitely way more of a trauma-informed provider – a relational provider. I really strongly emphasize the relationship with clients. That cannot be overstated. If anyone knows anything about me I hope it is that my relationships with my clients are the most important thing. If they don't trust me, they're not going to do anything or work on anything we talked about, which is fair – why would you?

I genuinely believe that my own experiences in therapy, and having had an eating disorder, have informed this, because the people I worked best with when I was a client were people who actually treated me like I was a person. [Katy is nodding vigorously] [Jess, wryly] I know, shocking! I also worked well with people who actually worked to get to know me, or worked to understand what was going on for me, instead of making blanket assumptions about what my experience was, which I think is a huge problem in the eating disorder world. There's a lot of assumptions.

I would say if there was a name for the type of therapy I do, it's relational therapy. This is just a fancy way of saying 'I really care profoundly for my clients and their experience', which is such a silly thing to say because it seems very basic! My work puts an emphasis on trauma-informed practices because, with eating disorders, we can work on behavioural stuff all day, but it's never just about behaviours. There's a whole lot of stuff under there. I do a lot of blending of things but, yeah, I'm a relational therapist.

Katy: That's very cool! It sounds like we work in quite a similar way.

Jess: Oh, cool!

Katy: I'm also remembering when I was a teenager and into my 20s, I had a lot of disordered eating stuff going on, and I was also a plus size, queer, chronically ill, neurodivergent person. I think if somebody had just been like, 'Okay, here's a CBT handbook!', I would not have done very well with this!

Jess: Just start hissing at them and run! [Katy laughs] Yeah, it's rough out there. I think there's not a lot of understanding that people don't fit into boxes, which means treatment is not going to be able to fit in a box, no matter how hard you try. Some things are just not going to work for people, and it's not their fault.

Katy: I know that, when I have clients coming to me and that's happened to them, they've been blamed for that – that they're not trying hard enough, that they're refusing the treatment...

Jess: That they're treatment resistant.

Katy: Yes! That they're treatment resistant.

Jess: [sarcastically] My favourite...!

We see this in the substance use world, and in some other parts of the mental health field, but I think it's really profound in eating disorder treatment. There's a lot of blaming people for not accessing health in the 'right way', or not recovering in the 'right way'. There's a stigma–harm–justification cycle. When a person is stigmatized because they have an eating disorder – or for any reason – then their eating disorder worsens. Depending on the person's identity, that can be even more pronounced. Then their treatment is compromised because of the stigma they've experienced, which means their outcomes are way worse, but they're blamed for the outcomes, so it's a really awful circle. Once you see it, it's hard to not see it, so I don't know how people don't see it. It gets pretty exhausting, actually.

Katy: I can imagine. How do you tend to deal with that exhaustion? How do you care for yourself while you do this job?

Jess: That's a question I've gotten throughout the years, so many times, and I think it's really hard to answer, in part because every year of the world that I have lived as a therapist has been worse than the last.

I remember when I first started my practice in Texas – it was 2018, and I can remember it being great. I thought, 'I got this! I'm good!' And then 2019 was just such a difficult year, professionally and personally, and I was like, 'Okay, it can only go up from here', and then 2020 was like, 'Oh, no...!'

Through all that, it's been really interesting to watch how clients behave, as a therapist, because I think there's so much less of a power differential now than there used to be. In part because clients know that we are living in real time with them through some of the worst moments of human history. They're living through a global pandemic, and watching lots of terrible stuff happen because of that, and I'm also seeing it. It's different when the client is just experiencing stuff in their own life; I'm not touched by it outside of me caring for them and wanting their life to be better. Whereas this, I think, really changed things. I'm sure we'll hear more about it as time goes on and research is done, but it does feel like it fundamentally changed the fabric of the therapy world because we're really in it with our clients. That, I will say, was challenging to manage.

That was a huge hindrance to my self-care because I felt like I was overcompensating a lot. It was like, 'I have to be the professional and I have to have it all together, and I have to make this work.' Which, spoiler alert, that was not great for my mental health!

I do like to do the traditional self-care things. I try to engage with things that make me happy. I try to take care of my physical health. I try to be outside if it's not 105 degrees.

I'm a big journaler – writing is a huge outlet for me. And reading. Those are two really big parts of my health care routine. I am also currently re-reading a series of fantasy novels and that's my favourite thing; I get really involved! It's like I'm there. I'm ten steps into that world a lot of the time.

I would say I try to do all those really general self-care things that get thrown around, the kind you see on social media, and sometimes they work and sometimes they don't. I do know without a doubt that, for me, therapy works, journaling works, reading works. Being with preferred people works. Being with my pets works. So, I try to do those things. Even then it can be difficult to not be exhausted, but it helps.

I'd say that the number one thing that allows me to take care of myself and deal with the exhaustion is going to my own therapy. I feel so fortunate that I can access therapy. When I was a younger therapist, really early on, I could not afford to see a counsellor with any regularity, so this has been such an amazing thing. I'm like, 'This is so luxurious! This is the greatest hour of my week! I love this! This is my time!' It's been an incredible experience, and I say this as someone that's gone to this therapist now for four years, but it doesn't even feel like that long.

Katy: What's it like for you to be a therapist and a therapy client?

Jess: It's been interesting. Being a therapist in therapy is its own unique experience.

Maybe also because someone allowed me to become a therapist at 25 years old. My frontal lobe was not even fully developed! [Katy laughs] You know, I still had so much stuff in my own life to work through because I was 25 – who doesn't? There was a lot I didn't understand. Plus, being a therapist, I really thought I was supposed to have it together, that it was very shameful for me to go to therapy, but I needed to go. I feel like that was a journey, finally getting to a place of, 'It's okay. Now this is non-negotiable. This is the greatest thing! There's nothing to be ashamed of.'

There is still a lot of shame and stigma about being a provider with any sort of mental health struggles. I think it has gotten better, but it is something that I look back on and feel sad about for my younger self, because I really was very strategic as a therapy client. I kept my cards real close to the chest in therapy, because I didn't want to get in trouble. I think that feeling was strong – 'I don't wanna get in trouble.' Whereas now I'll go to my therapist, and I'm like, [mischievous voice] 'Here! Hold this for me! I don't want to!' [Katy laughs] I think that really has changed so much for me, being able to have that, and to know that regardless of the week I have had I can go there and I will have a space for it, and I don't have to carry it by myself. That changed things for me in a major way.

Katy: Hearing you talk about this, it makes me remember that one of my favourite bits of self-care as a young therapist was going to therapy and learning that my therapist had a therapist, and letting that settle in! I think there's a stereotype that a therapist is supposed to be paragon of mental health. We're all supposed to have it together, as you said, but we're just human.

Jess: It's funny you say that. I have a client, and this was maybe earlier in our work together, and they just noted – it was very offhand, it wasn't meant to be insulting or anything – but they were like, 'You're a bit of a weirdo.' [Both laugh] I was not at a place in my journey where I was able to hear that without hearing an insult. I was a little fucking weirdo as a kid, and people teased me, so I was like [mimics holding back distress] but still I sat with it. I still see this client and it's now such a nice thought. Yeah, this person sees me for who I am as a person, not just as their therapist and, yeah, they know I'm a little fucking weirdo, and whatever, the world goes on. It's a nice thing.

Katy: There can be a real strength in that as well.

Jess: I think so, too. I think my weirdo-ness is a huge strength. I would not want to be a normie and a therapist! [Both laugh] It would not work for me or my clients.

Katy: I really get that. That brings me to my next question quite nicely! What drew you to working with queer clients with eating disorders?

Jess: It's funny – I don't think I was drawn to this. Like I said, I started working in this field as a very young person, and I knew that I wanted to work with eating disorders, but I didn't really have a huge plan outside of that. In fact, I think as a younger person and younger therapist, I didn't really consider that there were things beyond that – that I didn't just have to specialize in eating disorders, that there are pockets in this very large population of people that need more specific assistance. I think it was, more than anything, accidental. I think, over time, I just got a lot of referrals from folks who trusted me – but, at the time, I think they just thought I was an ally.

I am – and have been since age 19 or 20 – out as a queer person, but 'out' is relative. For a very long time I was hyper-hyper-feminine and I'd make it a joke. It was like I was in a girl costume all the time, like in a very normie cishet girl costume, so no one clocked me ever. And I am married to a cishet man. I always try to think about it from the place of like, yeah, it kind of sucks to have aspects of my identity be invisibleized, but that in and of itself is a privilege. That said, people were still referring queer clients to me, so there was at least some understanding. Even if queer clients didn't look at me and think that I was queer, they trusted that I could treat queer people, so that was nice. I always love that.

I also think that, a lot of the time, clients will find me and then they will clock me, which I think is because I dress differently now. My gender and queer expression is different than it was when I was younger, because I had a lot more fear when I was younger that I have less of now. I do think clients meet me and they're like, 'Oh, okay, you're one of us, great!' I think it's really entertaining that my clients sometimes know me better, or can assess me better, than I think they can. Clients are discerning and smart and can tell.

Katy: Maybe queer clients with eating disorders are drawn to you, instead of the other way round?

Jess: A super-important piece to note is that so many queer and trans people have eating disorders. Trans youth account for the largest population of people with eating disorders within the larger population. It's something like one in four people with eating disorders are also queer or trans. It's mostly trans youth, but queer and trans people are disproportionately affected compared to straight and cis people. No surprise there, frankly.

I was recently putting together a presentation and was reading some older literature, and articles from the early 2000s had hypotheses about how cis queer women would not experience eating disorders at all. I was laughing as I was reading it because it was so absurd. The argument is like, 'They're not impacted by the male gaze!' It sucks when eating disorders are reduced to the male gaze. Ultimately this research did find that queer women are experiencing eating disorders at the same rate as women who are not queer and, in fact, that bisexual women are experiencing eating disorders significantly more often. No wonder eating disorders are so underdiagnosed, especially in queer people. It is a curious thing and, again, I never would have thought about it when I was a younger clinician, because it just wasn't on my radar.

I also saw a lot of young people who were so disconnected from their bodies because they were teenagers with eating disorders. Many of them did not know about sexuality, frankly – that was not a conversation we were having. That changed over time, and that opened a whole different world for me, where I could talk about this as part of identity development. I feel really lucky to have done something so cool.

So this was something I stumbled into but, frankly, I don't know how people don't stumble here. If you work with eating disorders, I don't see how you're not also treating queer and trans people. Or, it does happen, and they're just not paying attention.

Katy: In your experience, what is it like to be a queer counsellor in America right now?

Jess: I currently live in Texas. I'm originally from the East Coast, and that is where I would prefer to be. Being in Texas and working with queer and trans folks is its own really frustrating experience

– not because of my clients, but because of the systems in place. I am very much an East Coaster, though. People can usually tell. I'm always very aggressive about it, like, 'I am not a Texan!' I really am not. [Katy laughs] No shade to Texans!

Katy: No, I get it!

Jess: But like I said, it's not me. I'm not one of that bunch.

What was probably most helpful in terms of really developing my skill set and having more queer clients is that I live in an area that is very progressive – which is hilarious because I live in Texas – but Austin is this unique little progressive bubble. Less so now, actually – sadly – than it was when I first moved here, but in 2017 this was like an oasis. I wasn't super happy to live in Texas but if I was going to end up in Texas, I am so grateful I have landed here. There are people here who are so openly queer and trans, and there's so much acceptance. There's no question about it. It's not the same as other places I've lived. Where I lived in New Jersey, before I moved, was very conservative, so it was a breath of fresh air when I first moved here and I saw a lot of queer and trans people living here. I think just by nature of that, I received a lot of referrals from people.

Again, I feel really fortunate, and also that 'fortunate' is the wrong word. I have privilege that does allow me to navigate the world and the field differently. I do think that is a really profound privilege I have, and I know that some of my queer and trans colleagues do not have that. I've tried to use that privilege for good, especially in the area I am in. If I can put myself in front of oppressed people, and try to make sure that they do have protection, I will.

Katy: I only want to ask this if you're comfortable answering. I'm curious what your own eating disorder recovery was like?

Jess: I never mind answering this question or speaking about my own experience of this. I am always mindful because, when I was going through having an eating disorder, and going through recovery, I was the pinnacle of the eating disorder stereotype. There are a lot of ways in which I had no experience of any pushback in my recovery process. Mind you, I think there's a lot of negative that I experienced that I'm like, 'If that was happening to me, what was happening for other people?' But I think, by and large, I was very fortunate, and I had access to a lot of things that other people didn't.

That said, I like to joke with people in my life that my recovery was a very feral process. I did a lot of finding my own way and doing my own thing. Even though I did have access to care, it was a little haphazard. I went to residential more than once but, for reasons unknown, they'd never set me up with step down care. Usually you go to residential, and then the hope is you 'step down' into partial or whatever. That did not happen for me at any point in my process. I look back on that and think it probably could have been helpful.

The last time I went to residential was when I was 19. Again, the same thing happened where I was launched out into the world and they were like, 'Let's see what happens.' I was like, 'I'm not doing this anymore. I'm not doing this again. I need to find my own way.' I created a hell of a roadmap in retrospect, but it had a lot of detours, as one does. A big part of my life after getting out of treatment was I worked at a... I'm not sure if you're familiar with what a diner is?

Katy: [laughing] Yes!

Jess: Okay! Sorry, I never know, 'cause it's such a...

Katy: It's very American.

Jess: Even when I moved to Texas, I was like, 'Do people know what that is?' Because it's such a New Jersey and New York thing.

Katy: We have them here in the UK as a novelty setting. Like, [bad American accent] 'Come check out this real American diner! We have those paper napkin dispensers and big milkshakes with two straws!'

Jess: I think that's kind of what it is everywhere else outside of New Jersey and New York! In New Jersey and New York, we're like, 'No no, this is real, we're taking ourselves very seriously.' Everywhere else it's like, 'This is very silly.'

But, anyway, I worked in a 24-hour New Jersey diner when I left treatment and it was probably the greatest thing that ever happened for my recovery, because I was surrounded by people who were, for the most part, a lot older than I was, and a lot of people who were also in recovery from substances. They surrounded me with love and really took care of me. In retrospect it was such an incredible experience – if I had not had that, I do not think I would have been set up as well as I was to keep going.

After that I went back to school and, again, launched myself head-first into my life with varying degrees of success. I would say that, over time, I learned to cope. I figured it out. It was not a good time, in part because so much was missed in my treatment – like being a queer person, being someone who is gender non-conforming, being neurodivergent. There are so many questions that I was never asked. There's so many aspects of my identity that were never identified.

It was difficult as a neurodivergent person, too. I got punished a lot in treatment for not following rules in the right way or pushing back on rules. I wasn't allowed to not want to do it. I got dropped a level – because treatment often uses a level system – for being too negative and asking too many 'inappropriate' questions. Things like that, right there – that was an opportunity. That could have given me so much information, but it wasn't available; that was just not part of treatment at that time.

There's a lot that I've learned about myself over the years that has allowed me to have a lot more compassion for 'younger me' in my recovery process, including all the identities I hold, and also acknowledging that trauma was a major part of my eating disorder. No one clocked that – no one thought that was important to mention.

There was also a lot of push for you, once you go to treatment, to be recovered, and you will be better, and you will also suffer from this for the rest of your life, and we'll need to be hypervigilant. I feel like that fucked with my head so much because, if I was struggling, it made it so hard to ask for help. There was also this lurking feeling that I was gonna have to deal with this until I die – so what was the purpose of asking for help? That was a lot to break out of, and something that I still struggle with. 'What's the point if I'm going to be dealing with this forever?'

Now I have more of an understanding that, yes, I am someone who has had an eating disorder, and I had an eating disorder for a very specific set of reasons. Just because I stopped using those behaviours and healed from that, does not mean that the reasons that created it went away. I wish someone would have told me that. It would have been so nice to know that, and to know that I would have to address those reasons. I have to work on them. I would have to heal from whatever it was that contributed to that. And that is work. I will do that work forever and now I'm okay with that. I am. I want to be the best version of myself. I do recognize that I will probably struggle with my mental health forever, because I'm a person who's had mental illness, and that's not a death sentence. It doesn't have to be a dark, hopeless experience. It can be a liberation.

Katy: What brought you to Health at Every Size (HAES) and fat liberation?

Jess: It's interesting, because I really had no concept of what Health at Every Size was, or what anything in that world was, until I was in graduate school. I was an avid Tumblr user – as one was in the early 2000s – and I stumbled upon this blog. It was run by a person named Jennifer and her handle on Tumblr was *fatsmartandpretty*. I remember that really rocked my world. I had never heard somebody use the word fat in a non-derogatory way. I pored over her blog and looked at everything she recommended to read, and it changed my life.

From there I read as much fat acceptance literature as I could get my hands on. I read *Lessons from the Fat-o-sphere* (Harding and Kirby, 2009); I read *Two Whole Cakes* (Kinzel, 2012); I read so many incredible books that I never would have had access to if I hadn't happened to stumble upon this person. It changed the way I viewed my own eating disorder because it gave me a lot more perspective that there's so much more than I am aware of. I mean, there's so much more than all of us are aware of, if you don't even know to look for it.

When I came into the field as an eating disorder therapist, Health at Every Size had not really been integrated yet, which is so funny to think about because now we've woven it into the fabric of eating disorder treatment. But when I started in 2015 Health at Every Size was seen as some kind of opposite to eating disorder treatment.

Katy: I saw that view in other mental health spaces, too.

Jess: I was kind of a squeaky wheel at times in the practice I worked for – I was like, 'No, I'm not doing that. I'm not saying that. I'm not recommending this person to do that. This doesn't make any sense.' In part it was because of the things I had read, and how they'd changed how I thought about things. It prevented me from causing a ton of harm that I didn't want to be causing, and it's been nice to see it be integrated into eating disorder treatment. I don't know how often it's adequately integrated, but I know there's some attempt, at least.

Over time I've just tried to stay as aware and knowledgeable as I

LGBTQ+ EATING DISORDER TREATMENT WITH JESS SPRENGLE

can. I want to know what fat liberationists are talking about. I think it's way more useful and helpful to me as a provider than it is to go to a training about Health at Every Size that's being taught by a thin person. There are times I teach about it, but we are not authorities. Thin people cannot be authorities in a movement that is not for us and does not benefit us in the same way. I try to acknowledge what I can and then I go to the source – the better source.

Katy: That's a cool way of looking at things. I'm interested, as well, to hear what your own journey with queerness has been like so far?

Jess: I feel like my life has almost cleaved in a few different places. I look back at me, age 19, and that's when it was a reality for me. I used the term bisexual at the time, because that just felt right to me. That was when it was real for me.

That said, though, I was thinking about this for way longer than that. I went through my journals from college and from high school and I could see it in those journals. It was interesting to watch my journey through that because, again, I was so lost; my queerness was lost to me, in part because I had a severe eating disorder. I also went to a Catholic school for 12 years.

Katy: That'll do it.

Jess: Yeah. Not very long after that, I met my now husband. We have been together for a very long time, 13 years now, and so there was not a whole lot of time between when I had this major revelation about myself and when I met this person who I ultimately married, and who I hope to spend the rest of my life with.

Katy: Awwww!

Jess: He's my person. He's a good one. So it is interesting to think about, because I had this experience, and then I almost caught myself off guard, where I was like, 'This can't possibly be real about me if I am marrying a man. If I am going to be in this relationship with this person, I just need to act like this is not real.' I did that for a very long time. I shoved it down and shoved it down, and it would pop back up at times, and then I'd have a crisis about who I was and what was happening.

I don't think I was really ready until I was here – shockingly, in Texas – and during the pandemic. I was like, 'Why do I hide this thing about myself? Why?' Because it's been real. It's been real for as long as I've been a person. I had just never let myself be open about it. I came out to a few people when I was in college, but it was like, 'What's the point of this, ultimately, if I'm gonna be in this relationship?' This time I was like, 'No one can tell me I'm not.' I think that exact thought dawned on me. 'No one can tell me I'm not. I can say this about myself, I know it's true, and no one can say I'm not.'

That was an experience I had, actually, when I was younger. I was dating somebody and I said to him, 'I think this is true about me.' And he was like, 'I think you just come up with this shit when you're bored.' My favourite part of this is that I forgot this interaction happened until within the last two years. Again, I'm an avid journaler – I have journals from, like, the fourth grade – and I read it in a journal within the last several years, and I was like, 'That couldn't have happened, could it?' And then I went back and looked at something else, and I had written it in more than one place. It definitely happened. People, ultimately, told me this isn't real, so I couldn't say it out loud. Not out loud.

And then I was like, you know what? Fuck this. My family members follow me on social media, and I think that was another part of it, where it was like, 'I don't wanna have to deal with this.' Ultimately, I was like, you know what? They don't have to look. They can unfollow me. They can go away.

The last several years have allowed me a little bit more space to actually explore what this part of myself means. This is an aspect of my life I've really not allowed myself to look at, because I didn't think I could, and now it's a very integral part of who I am. It's something all of the people who love me know about me. It's not something I hide. My clients know it about me. There's some grief there, and a very freeing feeling that I could have just done this all along.

It's still sometimes a little scary – obviously I share on social media, and on my website, that I identify this way, and that does come with potential for pushback, so that scares the part of me that was always like, 'You can't do this.' I'm actively bucking the part of me that couldn't tolerate that. It's like an exposure practice. It's an ongoing processing. I'm not sure where it'll take me, but I am not terrified of finding out any more in the way that I was when I was younger. It's more like, there might be something cool through this and I hope I find it.

Katy: This is a really cheesy therapist-y thing to say, but it sounds like you can protect that part of you now, the part that worries that people can take this away from you.

Jess: That's a very nice therapist thing to say! And it's true. I'm grateful to be an adult. It's such a silly thing to say! But it's like, oh, man, I do not have to deal with any of that shit anymore! Y'all can stay over there and exist in your own toxic soup. I don't have to be part of that and that is amazing. I can just be in my own soup, or whatever that is.

Katy: Yours is delicious soup! I love that.

Jess: It's non-toxic!

Katy: It's good soup! What good things bring you hope for the future?

Jess: The world is in such a terrible place, but I do work with a lot of young people – college age and early 20s – and I am always so heartened by how different Gen Z is compared with so many other generations, including millennials. There just seems to be this righteous passion for making the world a better place that is so inspiring to me. I listen to so many of them talk about the world and what they're going to do better. It's not even something they've had to dig too far to learn, it's just inherent. They just know that the world needs to be a better place and they can be part of that. That gives me a lot of hope for whatever might be coming, that this next generation of people can handle all of the ways in which the generations past have destroyed things. It is hard to have hope for the future, but that does give me a lot of hope for it. I feel relief that it's not just one big unending swathe of shit. There are people, children, who are able and willing to do better than all those people who've not had the power, but they do.

Also, cats. God, throw that in there. Cats give me hope for the future because there is no end to the number of cats that can exist and be around me.

Katy: Cats will keep going.

Jess: Yeah, they will. They will live on truly forever. They will outlive humanity. I believe that they're always gonna be here.

Katy: I love that. That gives me hope as well. I'll take that with me.

Jess: I haven't even thought about it until just this moment, but I believe it. I'm just thinking about my cats, and I'm like, yeah, it'll be fine.

Katy: I'm so glad that my cats don't know what capitalism is. Oh, they just get to be free!

Jess: I hope that I come back in another life as a well-taken-care-of cat, because that seems amazing. My cats are living the life, they really are. I was saying to my husband yesterday, cats are such good role models for eating disorder recovery because they're so discerning and particular about food. They don't want to eat something that's not gonna taste good. They want to enjoy their experience. Also, because cats are so picky about food, we humans like to cater to their every need, as if this were our one goal. As if my one purpose in life is to make sure that Nugget, one of my cats, has his food mixed perfectly. Otherwise he will not eat it. Like, my god, I did not evolve for this – but, apparently, I did.

Katy's post-interview thoughts

Jess's energy around providing good care to their clients and themself through dark times was infectious – I left this interview feeling buoyed and hopeful. As a person-centred therapist, I particularly loved hearing about Jess's commitment to relational depth and safety for their vulnerable clients, therapeutic foundations that have timelessly proven to be the backbone of good psychological care (Rogers, 1957) and that can keep us working towards wellness despite the odds (Abbate-Daga *et al.*, 2013). I also appreciated the reminder that the ideal of therapists having it all together is an illusion that we don't have to play up to, especially as our congruence and humanness often helps with client connection (Turmaud, 2021).

If you'd like to know more

@thecrankytherapist on Instagram. This is Jess's Instagram account, which is full of wisdom and therapeutic memery. It's definitely worth a follow.

I'm Triggered podcast, by Megan O'Laughlin and Jess Sprengle. Jess's podcast, which started at the end of 2023. It explores two therapists' takes on triggers and glimmers in movies and TV. www. imtriggeredpod.com

Lessons from the Fat-o-sphere: Quit Dieting and Declare a Truce with Your Body, by Kate Harding and Marianne Kirby, 2009. A book mentioned by Jess as being helpful in their early understanding of fat acceptance. The book explores body image and outlines ways to connect with your body through fat acceptance, intuitive eating, and HAES ideals.

Two Whole Cakes: How to Stop Dieting and Learn to Love Your Body, by Lesley Kinzel, 2012. Another classic book that Jess read at the beginning of their fat acceptance journey. This book takes a look at how the media encourages harmful ideas around food, shame, and body size, and explores body acceptance and confidence.

Decolonizing Wellness: A QTBIPOC Centered Guide to Escape the Diet Trap, Heal Your Self-Image, and Achieve Body Liberation, by Dalia Kinsey, 2022. One of my top picks when it comes to fat-positive and LGBTQ+ body work, this book offers an exploration of how to offer yourself and your body compassion in the face of oppression and shame.

Queer Body Power, by Essie Dennis, 2022. This is another recommendation from me! This book looks at fat acceptance through a radical queer perspective.

Queer Dreaming with Rae

An introduction to Rae

Rae (she/her) is a queer, gender-expansive, person-centred, and experiential psychotherapist and supervisor in the UK with expertise in dreamwork, different facets of therapeutic growth, exploration of power dynamics, and working with the transpersonal. She wanted to be introduced here by her nickname, Rae, instead of the full name she practises under. Rae and I trained together in person-centred psychotherapy, and we remain friends even as she joyfully raced ahead of me in her studies.

In my own work as a psychotherapist, more and more of my queer clients have started bringing their dreams – and nightmares – into our sessions. Poor quality sleep is common in LGBTQ+ people (Fredriksen-Goldsen *et al.*, 2013; Blosnich *et al.*, 2014; Chen and Shiu, 2017; Harry-Hernandez *et al.*, 2020), and it made me wonder how dreams and nightmares show up for queer people and what those dreams mean to our community.

Working with dreams and transpersonal connection is a long-studied area of psychotherapeutic work, made popular by Sigmund Freud (Freud, 1899), Carl Jung (Jung and Jaffé, 1963), and Abraham Maslow (Maslow, 1968) from the early 1900s. This work was carried on in new ways by counselling contemporaries who look beyond the personal in therapy into ways in which we are connected to others and to the universe as a whole. Exploring our relationship with the transpersonal in therapy can be ground-breaking, whether we feel connected to the spiritual or not (Maslow, 1968). As we explore dreams as a way of being spoken to by our bodies – and perhaps more – we can start to hold our dreams as a potential for communal and personal healing (Koch, 2012).

I knew that Rae was going to be the person to speak to about queer dreaming. I remember Rae becoming more interested in dreams shortly after she finished her person-centred training, and her expertise in dreamwork has always been exciting to chat about. I experience Rae as being quick witted and fast flowing, while also prioritizing time to slow down and thoughtfully experience the present moment. She once complimented me by saying my therapeutic style is like 'being grounded by warm stone' and, likewise, I tend to experience her way of being as like being grounded by a cool river. Our interview felt a little like that, too – expansive, exciting, embodied, and full of mutual invitations to share.

Rae's interview

Rae: You can call me Rae. I'm a psychotherapist in terms of what I do for a living, and I've got a particular interest in dreams and spirituality. For me, dreams, spirituality, and psychotherapy are all one tree with different branches.

I love sci-fi too, and I love music. In the last nine months or so I've also massively got into exercising – not with any fitness goals, but just being in my body, moving and dancing. I feel like this past year has been the first time I've felt really, really safe to sink into being in my body, and enjoy my body, and move my body in ways that feel good for me.

Katy: What kind of exercise, and what kind of dancing, have you been doing?

Rae: I've just been dancing a lot at home with the music turned up! With exercising, I've been doing weightlifting, which is making me feel strong in my body. There's been a bit of running, and swimming, and walking. This is totally new for me, because I had such a disorganized relationship with my body, so moving in it has felt strange.

I also love singing. That feels like it fits in along with the exercise. Singing has been something I've been doing more of in the past couple of years.

Katy: The last time I saw you in person, you'd just started singing lessons! That sounds like it's been really grounding for you. I'm thinking about how singing and intentional movement both involve a lot of breath work, as well.

Rae: 100%! That's part of how it links with the exercise – it's about being in your self, isn't it? It's about being. Singing means using your own voice, but it also feels quite transcendent in some way.

Katy: What kind of therapy do you practise?

Rae: I work with adult individuals in my little therapy room here in the Midlands (UK). I work online and in person.

I was trained – with you! – as a person-centred and experiential psychotherapist. I always see that as my foundation in my therapy work. My base is really about wanting to get to know the person, who that person is, so I can follow them and meet them where they're at. Holding their well-being is the focus of the therapy, so I learn what well-being means to that person and follow on that journey with them.

I aim to practise a kind of therapy where I'm supporting the soul of the person to be in life, in whatever way that looks like for that individual. When I say 'soul', I mean that kind of authentic essence of a person, that uniqueness.

Katy: How did you become interested in therapeutic dreamwork?

Rae: I trained to be a therapist and finished around 2015/2016. In those two or three years after that, I had some really big dreams. I don't think I'd ever paid attention to my dreams before then, apart from, you know, when you might say to somebody, 'Oh, I had a really weird dream last night: I was being chased by a giant cushion,' or something like that! I'd never paid attention to my dreams until I started having a series of dreams that somehow felt big – and by that, I mean they left a profound imprint upon waking. These were dreams that left me feeling like they had been more than just the kaleidoscope of my psyche, more than my brain throwing up what had happened in the last week. It felt like there was something deeper happening, so I started writing my dreams down in a dream diary.

I then had an opportunity to study dreams in depth, in relation to psychotherapy. I wanted to learn more about the crossover between therapy and dreaming, so I started a course in dreamwork. That really unlocked a whole other layer of it. I was part of a great group of five people who met every week for two years and shared dreams, and worked with dreams in a particular way. That group lifted the lid on a whole new world that I'd never encountered before. That work meant that I started to see things through a slightly different lens – or, maybe, it was that it gave me another lens to add to the lenses that I already looked at myself and my clients through.

All of this changed how I processed clients bringing dreams to sessions. I think I didn't used to know how to respond to that, and I would maybe just listen in the way that I would listen to anything that a person shared with me, but I didn't really have any kind of tools or insights around dreams. I didn't know how to go deeper with the dreams of clients.

So it was sort of twofold – I had the personal journey of working with dreams, which then fed into my practice. It all supported me to be able to journey with my clients and their dreams, and work with what those dreams might mean for my clients.

Katy: So interesting! As you're talking about that, I'm remembering how important that dreamwork group was to you back then.

I'm also remembering way back when we were studying, and we were doing triad work where I was in the role of the therapist and you were in the role of the client. As the client, you talked about a nightmare that you'd had that had been bothering you.

Rae: Oh my gosh, I've not thought about since we did that! I remember that, but I can't remember what the dream was about that I was sharing with you.

Katy: You were the last person alive in the apocalypse, and everything was just a blasted landscape, and you were horrified and panicking.

Rae: Wow! That says so much about how I was feeling at the time! I think it's incredible that you remember that, and also I feel really relieved that you remember it so clearly. It's interesting that the ripples of meaningful dreams had been there, and they obviously were there enough for me to share that with you in that practice session that we had together. I guess I've been doing this work for a while, even when it hadn't consciously begun.

It's my experience that dreams always contain some magic in them that seems to move us towards growth rather than just darkness. Even nightmares, as crazy as that might sound. I think nightmares are something within us trying to be worked through, coming into consciousness to be let go or to be transmuted in some way.

Katy: It sounds like consciously beginning this work with your dream group taught you a lot about therapy work and also about yourself?

Rae: 100%. It was the group work that drew the line in the sand, that this is part of my life and the way that I see the world now. It taught me how to be able to relate to my dreams.

I don't know if you've ever done tarot cards with friends or anything, but there's that experience where you're turning something over and everyone's like: 'What do you see in this?', 'I see this there,' 'That's so interesting, because I can see something else, too.' Through that process of circling around the dream, there's something that happens where we come to meet the meaning for ourselves. There is meaning, but there's a journey to go on to find the meaning, and the journey creates the meaning, too, if that's not too paradoxical.

Katy: I love existential meaning making!

Rae: In the group I learned that everybody's dreams have a particular signature. It's like there's a unique language, almost, that different people's dreams use. There's some benefit in sharing an isolated dream with somebody, be that in therapy or with friends, but being part of the dream group also showed me that hearing lots of an individual's dreams taught me that unique language for each person over time. I could recognize that this was that person's dream, because their dreams had themes that reoccur, or there's a quality to their dreams that nobody else in the group had. It's a total privilege to follow another person's dreams over time. Everyone's way of dreaming had a uniqueness.

Katy: I've never thought about dreams as being that kind of personal before, which is really weird, because of course they are!

Rae: Yeah, they're really personal! I think that spirit of uniqueness kind of relates to queerness, too.

Katy: How do you think your queerness and your dreamwork interlink?

Rae: For me, there's an intersection between looking at my dreams and looking at my own queerness. There's something about my queer identity which is about being able to be in contact with lots of parts of myself, and being able to be in the freedom of that – to be unique and authentic, in my own way. Part of my relationship to my queer identity has been realizing that the label of 'queer' nicely holds some aspects of myself that maybe can't be contained anywhere else in me.

I think the link with dreams, and how dreams have maybe crossed over with that, is that dreams can be a free-for-all in terms of how you process yourself. When we're sleeping, there's no input from other people. I see it as our pure creative imagination that's generating these worlds and possibilities. Your imagination might be influenced by things that you've experienced – things in popular culture, for example – but in terms of what's generated, it's totally from the uniqueness of each individual person. So, when exploring my dreams, it's often hard to separate it out and say which bit relates to being queer and which bit's related to something else but, in a way, it's a perfect landscape to explore personal identity and what different dreams mean to different people.

For me and my own identity I've got a good example. I had a 'big' dream a while ago that I was in a minibus in America. I was part of some sort of touring group. We stopped at a service station, and I went to the toilets, and there were male and female toilets that were gendered with the usual kind of sign. In between those signs – in the gap between the two doors – there was a symbol that indicated 'no gender' to me, and it had a border around it that was neon and moving. I went through that door. I went through that gap in between, and met a person in there, and had an encounter in this space. It was almost like an old school doctor's room. I had an interaction, a dialogue, with this character that was on the other side of the door. What that dream unlocked for me, personally, is that it helped me to identify within myself the part of me that's beyond being seen as 'this' or 'that'. I kind of don't even want to use the word 'non-binary', because putting a label on it feels like it then limits the experience again. That dream unlocked my being able to connect to the conditioning that gender expectations have brought in my life, and some of the experiences that connect to that, and where I have felt limited by them. That was a dream that I took to this dream group that I was a part of. Exploring it with others was an unleashing – there was a kind of freedom in talking it through. Somebody within the group supported me to go back into the dream and dialogue with this person on the other side of the 'middle way' door. It was a very heart-centred opening up for me.

I also remember when you and I met up for a day out in York (in England), and we were talking about dreams, and you said you were excited to chat about queer dreaming with me for this book, and that was because I'd shared with you that I'd had a dream about meeting Elton John at a Christmas party! [Both laugh] Elton took me shopping, and we were buying these glittery birthday cards. I think I maybe dream of queer icons more than a person who doesn't identify as queer. For me, there's a real kind of humour in the characters that might show up in my dream, and I would say a lot of my dream characters maybe are queer. There's something about dreams that can defy the norms of the life that we live in, so in a dream it's perfectly normal, isn't it, to be finding queer doors and chatting with queer icons.

This actually reminds me of another dream of mine. In this dream I met a guy at an airport, and he's wearing a tweed dress and he's got a beard, and he looked great. Entering back into day-to-day waking life, we might come up against those conditioned ideas that dressing that way is not okay, whereas in the dream world, it's such a wonderful, regular part of things.

Katy: That has me thinking about how queerness can be especially congruent in a dream world.

Rae: It's just a thing that's happening. There's no external gaze that limits that world. This connects to what I was saying earlier, about how these aspects are totally from the world of the dreamer, unless there is a figure in your dream that's trying to pass judgement. There's just you – there's your world that's unfolding in the dream.

Katy: What have you found particularly interesting or different around dream interpretation with queer people?

Rae: For some of my clients, bringing dreams to therapy can be a way to work through some themes around their queer identity, queer relationships, and queer experiences. We can ask questions like – was your dream self in line with your waking identity? How did you feel in the dream world when you could just be without agenda? How do you feel in life where you are gendered, compared to how you were gendered in the dream? How did it feel to be able to be in the dream world and have relationships with multiple people, and what did that activate in you compared to your waking life where there's more limitation?

Katy: It sounds like quite a safe way of working with things.

Rae: Exactly. Again, it's such a privilege and a joy. You're working with the beautiful unique dream world of a person, and the word that comes to my mind is something about 'cherishing' – cherishing that uniqueness of the person. When a person brings their dream to you, there's no space for you to say, 'Well, that shouldn't be like that. Are you sure you dreamed that? Are you sure that's what you felt in the dream?' That person made that world. There's no question that this is what this person is bringing to you.

In terms of differences in dreamwork between people who identify as queer and those who don't, I think the themes that arise can end up being different. I'm making a generalization based on my experience here, so I feel like I want to tread carefully because I can't say this is the same for all therapists or all queer people who work with their own dreams, but – in my experience – there are some themes around identity, how they might show up in the world, and how that might be experienced and perceived that tend to come up in a different way with queer people. For a person who's processed their identity in a cisheteronormative way, those questions about identity might be less obvious in their dreams. For queer clients, you might be working with more psychological content or emotions around trauma and oppression, which might show up in their dream world. Obviously all of this is variable for everybody, but I think maybe the differences in dreaming might be around how we feel into aspects of our identity.

Katy: This really has me reflecting on a dream that I had last night!

Rae: Do you want to share? I'd love to hear it. I would love to listen.

Katy: I'm feeling a little bit of shame about it, which is so interesting, but it would be great to share!

In last night's dream I was getting married to the boy that I dated as a teenager, who continued to mess me around into my 20s. We got married in a ceremony that was not my style at all. It got to the evening of our wedding day and he was like, 'Actually, I don't think this relationship is gonna work out for me. I don't think you're the right person for me. I'm just gonna head off.' I was horrified, like, 'Why couldn't you have told me this before I got married to you?', and he was like, 'I don't know. Anyway, bye!' I was sat on the floor crying. And Lucy, my actual wife, came to find me. I was like, 'I so wish that I had married you instead,' and she said, 'But honey, we are married.' I was like, 'What?!' And she said, 'Yes, we're married, and we love each other.' I was like, 'Oh, thank god! Oh, what a relief! I'm so glad that I'm married to you!' [Both laugh] And then I woke up!

Rae: Wow! That journey sounds almost like a dream within a dream, in that you had to process that these awful things had happened, and then you had the realization that that's not actually real, that it's okay. How did you feel in the different parts of the dream?

Katy: When I was getting married in the dream, I felt like it wasn't right. It didn't feel good. I felt nervous about getting married, about being married. Something felt very wrong, like a weighted dread. When this person decided they didn't really like me, I felt very sad, very worried, and very rejected. And then, when dream-Lucy found me, I felt really, really relieved and I felt this huge wave of affection for her. Then, when I woke up, I was just kind of like, 'That was weird!' [Both laugh]

Rae: What a journey! There's this movement from something that felt tense and ill-fitting in to that feeling of relief and joy. I love that!

One of the things that I'm curious about is the people in your dream. If we go with the idea that the characters in our dreams are symbolizing a part of ourselves and our dream worlds, I'm wondering what parts of yourself Lucy and this guy from your past might represent? This is just one perspective – one tool – and not necessarily the truth, so this may or may not resonate with you and this dream, but who are they to you, in the dream, if they were bits of you?

Katy: When I'm not specifically dreaming about Lucy or our relationship, she'll still just kind of pop up sometimes. Often, when she does, I'll have a moment of relief – like, 'Phew, Lucy's here. I'm safe now. It's gonna be okay.' So I think Lucy was there as a safety thing.

It's interesting, as well, because the kind of tenseness that I felt when I was getting 'straight dream-married' to this guy felt quite like how I actually felt in that actual relationship, when I was trying really hard not to be queer. When I fell for this guy, it was a relief that that meant I was 'just a normal straight girl after all'. I wasn't, obviously, but at the time there was a relief that I'd finally fallen for a boy instead of a girl, and that I could stop worrying about what those other queer parts of me meant.

Rae: I feel quite moved. There's both a spirit of sadness in me, but also joy at you moving through to a period of your life where you feel that you can be you. I can hear the layers of that in this dream – when you want something because you don't want to be different, and the undercurrent being that something really doesn't feel right about it.

Katy: I remember, when I was getting dream-married, I was very much dressed 'like a girl', too, instead of like myself. I didn't feel comfortable at all. I wanted to take the dress off.

Rae: So something really didn't fit, literally!

Katy: Right!

Rae: It's so interesting that this dream-guy told you he wasn't the one for you – which always is sad and confusing – but that left room for the reality of your wife, your person who makes you feel safe. What a beautiful resolution within the dream.

The endings of our dreams are so interesting. Sometimes we might remember a snippet of a dream that just ends at the tense point of the dream. Sometimes we don't know if the dream actually ends there, or if there's more we're missing or don't remember. I think what you shared is really beautiful, because it shows the resolution of you coming back to your life and to your true self. It's like part of you knew that we were speaking today and wanted to throw you a perfect example!

Katy: Love that for us! Thanks, brain!

Rae: It's lovely. Thanks for sharing that dream.

Katy: You're very welcome. Thank you for sharing your dreams with me, too!

Rae: Here's another good example for you. I recently had a dream where me and a group of people were checking out the remains of this house that had burned down, and it turned into a party. I met this guy there, whose wife was also at the party, and the guy asked if I wanted to get together with him. I asked him, 'Is your wife okay with that?' He called his wife over so I could meet her, and she was like, 'Sounds great! Go have fun, you two! Off you go!' This dream feels connected to my queerness because of its sense of relationship fluidity, and in my accepting that within myself in terms of heteronormative identities versus queer identity. If I'd had that dream ten years ago I might have been like, 'What the fuck? [Both laugh] It's so wrong to get with somebody else's partner!' Whereas, in the dream, there's this lovely interaction where there's consent from the wife and everyone's happy. It doesn't feel like shocking subject matter to me. There are several layers in there that feel symbolic of aspects of myself that have shifted.

Katy: I love that dream-you wanted everyone's consent, as well!

Rae: Yeah, it was a good dream! [Both laugh]

Katy: My understanding of dreamwork is that it often involves ideas about the transpersonal – that we're all bigger than just ourselves. How do you hold the transpersonal and the spiritual in your therapy work?

Rae: That word – spiritual – I guess it can feel quite [makes a spooky noise] to some people. Spirituality could mean so many things but, for me, it means the journey of becoming who I truly am, and engaging in things that support me to become more of who I truly am. Spirituality is about the things that make me feel closer to who I truly am, but also to who we are, in a sense of who we are collectively and how we are all connected in some ways. In that way spirituality and the transpersonal can be huge parts of therapy and dreamwork. I think that's why your dream is so beautiful to me, because it shows that spiritual journey towards queer congruence so well.

I wonder if it's also about the journey that we've been on in Western therapy, too, in terms of dreamwork within psychotherapy. That has been heavily influenced by Carl Jung, who formally introduced transpersonal ideas into Western psychology, with archetypal themes and the symbolism that often happens in dreams. In the transpersonal community that I'm connected with now, dreamwork is a massive part of that mode of being a therapist, and so dreams are a big part of how we practise therapy.

Katy: Do you think there are transpersonal aspects of queerness?

Rae: Absolutely, I do. I think queerness and the transpersonal are kind of the same, in a way. Transpersonal, to me, means more than the individual, so we're talking about that collective world that we might inhabit, not just physically but also in other dimensions. There are ways in which we might be connected that aren't about our physically being next to each other, and I think that's a huge part of being in queer community, for me. This is just for me, again – each person who identifies as queer is obviously going to be different, and for every single person queerness and queer community is going to feel different – but, for me, queerness is about both individual and collective identity.

I guess another way to phrase this question could be, 'Is queerness spiritual?' There can be spirituality in identifying as queer, or maybe even going on a journey with that question. Figuring out that relationship to queerness is, for me, a spiritual journey. Finding your authentic self can be a spiritual journey. Those queer questions – who are you, and how do you want to express yourself in life? – can be spiritual. I think that we're definitely deeply connected in asking and answering those questions.

There's something about being part of queer communities where I can bring more of myself, just naturally. I feel like more of me is present in any given environment that might feel like a safe queer space for me. I think that speaks to the safety of being able to connect with the authenticity of our deeper nature, and that being in community can make that so much easier. Being together helps us to be more fully whole.

Katy: What else helps you to feel whole as a queer person?

Rae: Again, dreamwork has been a tool that's helped me and my discovery of my queerness. It's been a tool that's helped me on my journey of understanding myself as a queer person, and being able to be comfortable in my inner world in ways that then allow me to express that externally in my life.

Having queer therapy with a queer therapist has also helped. It's not just about seeing a therapist who is queer, for me, but working with a queer therapist who also integrates that in their work in a way that feels very supportive, nurturing, not intrusive, and not passive. Having queer friends helps me to feel like myself, as well as having safe spaces where I can just be myself.

Maybe not so much now, but there was a period in my life where it was helpful to look for queer community on social media, and in films and things like that, so I could absorb aspects of culture and up-to-date conversation. It was helpful to see queer figures who are out there on social media, and to see queer films and take in queer stories.

Katy: Is there anything you'd really like queer people to know, or to think about, in terms of mental health?

Rae: If you can have connection within the queer community in some way, that for me feels so important. If I think about mirroring – we need that mirroring, don't we? We need to see ourselves out there. This is something that my therapist introduced to me – they talked about the need for queer mirroring. If a person is queer and raised by heterosexual cisgender parents, then the parents might not be attuned in a way that supports the queerness within their child. We see that continuing to play out for queer adults in a society where heterosexuality and being cisgender are the expected norm. I would say to seek out queer mirroring for your own mental health, so that you know queerness keeps existing in the world. If you exist in a world where a part of you, or parts of you, are not mirrored back to you, how do these parts get to flourish? How do these parts get to live free from shame, free from the restrictions that can sometimes feel so overwhelming? That would be my big advice for queer people

– finding one's community for mirroring. I know that this kind of safety is not always possible for everybody, but seeking out people who are safe, and bases that feel safe, can make so much difference to how you feel.

Now that I'm thinking about it, I wonder if Lucy being there as the safe person in your dreams is connected to queer mirroring? That idea that, when you're together, you're both safe to be yourselves?

Katy: Thinking about safety, community, congruence, and queer mirroring all together has me thinking about Sam Hope's Web Model. That's the idea that, whenever we meet somebody, we create a relational thread. The more that we have in common, or the more community that we share, the more threads are going to be intact between us. If we meet people who don't get it, even if they're not being mean, that thread is going to be weak, or chafed, or non-existent. The more friendships that we have with people, the more we feel seen and heard, and the more understood we are, the stronger and safer we feel. When we belong to an oppressed group of people it can be hard to create good threads with others, but the webs we do create can really hold us. It makes sense that those threads would show up in our dreams, too!

Is there any advice you'd give to people who want to pay more attention to their own dreams?

Rae: Delight in your dreams. Spend time with your dreams. This goes back to this idea that I hold, which is that our dreams come from the creative core of ourselves, from a deeper part of ourselves. Dreams form on the fringe of consciousness and unconsciousness, and paying attention to what's there can be a beautiful journey of discovery. Nobody gets to tamper with your dreams – they're purely you!

As a tool for deepening your connection with yourself, I would recommend working with your dreams by writing them down and processing them, by yourself and with people you trust. Something that I sometimes do is I draw something from my dream, even. I'd recommend this to anybody.

Katy: I'm going to start doing this. I'm so jazzed about dreams now!

Rae: I'm still part of a dream group, but it's a different group to before. There's four of us in the group, and we're all queer. We all identify as queer in different ways. For me, that's one of my webs! Although our queer identity isn't the focus of why we meet, that's a natural part that's in there as we're sharing dreams. We have a shared understanding, so there's more of an attunement as to how different bits of our dreams might resonate in terms of queer identity and queer aspects of self. The power that holds is huge, just by virtue of sharing our worlds with one another. It's just a beautiful thing to do.

I think research around dream sharing has shown that, through sharing dreams, empathy is increased. Our skill for empathizing with other people is increased through sharing our dreams and listening to the dreams of others.

Katy: From everything that we've talked about today, that makes a lot of sense. Sharing dreams involves a lot of different ways of seeing the other person's world.

With that in mind, how would you recommend other therapists work with their clients around their dreams?

Rae: You don't have to have any specific tools to get started. There seems to be some magic that gets unlocked just through talking about dreams and people sharing interest about them. Showing interest in your clients' dreams means showing interest in their inner worlds.

The content of dreams can sometimes be really difficult to share, including with our therapists. Sometimes it can be difficult, and sometimes wonderful, and then other times it can be outright bizarre. It might not always be easy to share some dreams, but I think all of our dreams are valuable in some way or another, so I think it's always worth following your client's lead when it comes to dreams. I think my willingness to hold space for that is not hidden from my clients, because it always energizes me to talk about dreaming, which makes therapy a safe space for them to bring their dreams even when it's hard. Even if their dreams are just the wacky ones, engaging with that can be a way to show your clients they have no bad or boring parts. It means inviting your client to bring something so precious to the table, like a work of art from the core of themselves.

Katy's post-interview thoughts

When I left this interview I felt energized about exploring dreams as a means of connection to others and myself. Although it's probably common sense that dreams are extremely personal to us, it had never really sunk in for me before that dreams are both a unique personal language and a possible means of cultural connection. My conversation with Rae was a joyful reminder that queer people are connected through imagery, congruence, culture, authenticity, freedom, and mirroring in conscious and unconscious ways. It's lovely to think that queerness is more than individual in a way that makes anything possible.

I've been trying to journal about my dreams more since this interview, and it's been interesting to see different aspects of how I talk to myself while my brain is completely self-directed. It also turns out my dreams are really queer – go figure!

If you'd like to know more

The Dream Research Institute. This offers therapeutic dreamwork training and workshops, dream groups, resources, and further research. www.driccpe.org.uk

This Is Why You Dream, by Rahul Jandial, 2024. This book provides a more modern look at dreaming, written by a neurosurgeon. Rigorously cited, it explores how the biological, psychological, sociological, and personal all play into the alchemy of dreams.

Sam Hope's *Web Model.* In this interview I mention the Web Model when talking to Rae about queer connection. The Web Model is a fascinating anti-oppressive relational framework, exploring how we connect to others – or not – when we experience minoritization. I first read about it in Hope's book *Person-centred Counselling for Trans and Gender Diverse People: A Practical Guide* (2019).

Balancing Parts with Viv

An introduction to Viv

This collaborator asked me to pick a pseudonym for her, and I chose 'Viv'. I felt it suited her, and I'd also just finished reading *Bookshops and Bonedust* by Travis Baldree, in which an orc named Viv goes on emotionally healing sapphic adventures by the sea. Although this Viv is not much like Orc-Viv, it just felt right.

Viv (she/her) is a white, disabled, gender-expansive lesbian currently practising psychotherapy in the north of England. She was one of the only out queer people studying in my original cohort of our person-centred psychotherapy course, and we've remained friends past that training process. She also finds some of her own therapeutic peace by making pottery, of which I'm the delighted owner of a few pieces. Her therapy practice centres on young LGBTQ+ clients and survivors of childhood sexual abuse, often using 'parts work' as a therapeutic tool.

Parts work involves addressing the needs of your different configurations of self (Mearns, 1999; Mearns and Thorne, 2000; Cooper *et al.*, 2004) – that is, looking at your different inner parts, like your inner child or your inner critic, to find out what they're trying to tell you about yourself. LGBTQ+ people often experience adverse childhood events (Lowary, 2022; Jones and Worthen, 2023), including childhood sexual abuse (Capaldi, Schatz, and Kavenagh, 2024), so parts work that helps us reconnect to younger parts of our identities can be an especially important and interesting part of queer-centred trauma therapy.

I'm always excited to talk about parts work, gender nonconformity, and different kinds of queer person-centred therapy practice, so I knew I wanted to interview Viv for this project. It took some light coaxing, as she was anxious that she wasn't interesting enough to take part but – as you're about to learn – of course, she is. I really appreciate her steadfast energy and her gentle joie de vivre, and interviewing her was heartfelt and moving.

Viv's interview

Viv: I'm going to be open about some things, and some things I'm holding back, because they're not my story to tell.

So, my pronouns are she/her. I work in private practice as a therapist, and I also work as a sessional counsellor both with a charity supporting survivors of childhood sexual abuse, and with young LGBTQ people. I grew up in a small Midlands (UK) market town in the 1960s. The 1960s, 70s, and 80s were my formative years. It was very different to now, obviously, in terms of LGBTQ life.

In terms of my sexuality, I'm a lesbian. In terms of my gender, I sort of sit in some grounds that I don't know ever quite gets described by others. I'm content describing myself as female – that feels alright – and sometimes I can do a bit of femininity, especially if I can muck it up a bit. This might come in later, but you know that bow tie and nail varnish combination – that's what I enjoy. It's like, 'Right. You've got some ideas about me? Sort that out! What do you think? Because actually, I like both of those things!' That's probably about as clear as I get, really.

Katy: I love that kind of energy. I'm thinking back to when I was trying to find words that described what being non-binary meant to me, and finding words like 'genderfuck'.

Viv: Yeah! I'll just do what I like. I do what interests me, and I dress however I want, and I don't really care if they're normally categorized one way or the other. Why should that make a difference? I can reject all that. I just don't see how it really applies to me as I am. Although, once you're out in society, there's a bit more pressure to put on a performance, but I try not to do that too much.

Katy: What was it like, to grow up LGBTQ+ in 1960s and 70s England?

Viv: I don't remember any positive aspects to being LGBTQ then. There were no positive role models, so that was hard. Once I was in senior school there was one physical education teacher who was probably a lesbian, but she wasn't out, because nobody was going to be out. Other than that, for me, there was nothing positive anywhere. Nothing at all. I had this embodied sense, when I was doing my therapy dissertation and trying to look back at what might have been in the papers at the time, that the only lesbians you'd ever read about in the papers were when a lesbian had murdered her partner. That was kind of it, so there was nothing to read about people like me other than salacious 'axe murderer' articles – and we were reading *The Guardian*, never mind the lurid papers. It was completely devoid of any sort of way of knowing anything about what being a lesbian even was. I would say that pretty much carried on through my early life.

My mum and dad both grew up in Ireland. Now that I look back, we weren't a regular family like the families around us. I've never really known what 'roots' meant, which is another curiosity in my life. I was quite studious and quiet as a child; I was the sort of child who was very helpful. I guess, now, with my psychotherapeutic understanding, that's how I made sure that I was liked. I would help people with schoolwork and help at home. My mum was ill on and off quite a lot, so I was probably a bit adultified. It was too soon, in terms of the household chores and responsibilities – there was quite a lot that ended up on me because my dad was a teacher, and he was busy working and following his interests. It was quite gendered.

Even though there were those strict gender roles in my life, my parents were really understanding when I was gender non-conforming as a child. It's funny, because I can remember my sister and I getting little cowboy outfits when we were little. I'm the eldest, and we're both tomboys – that's not really ever changed for me! I think my mum found it a bit harder later on, that I kept being a tomboy. I could turn on being feminine now and then, but it wasn't something that I'd normally bother doing – I didn't really see the point.

Katy: We were two of the openly LGBTQ+ trainees in our original therapy training group. What was your experience of that like?

Viv: I don't know if I was worried about it beforehand. Honestly, I don't remember. I must have thought about it. But then, in the very first session, you had to write something about yourself on a piece of paper and people had to guess which fact belonged to which person. I thought, 'I might as well do it now and find out what I'm up against here', so I wrote, 'I am gay.' Then people were trying to figure out who all the things belong to. I thought that was fascinating.

Katy: I remember there were two people who wrote some kind of iteration of 'I am gay,' and someone guessed that I had written one of them. And I was like, 'Yes, I am! But, no, I didn't!' I wrote that I once scuba dived through a helicopter.

Viv: I remember being heartened that somebody else had written the same thing. That was great. It was such an interesting exercise in the group, wondering who would write each thing. I remember being amazed by your scuba diving fact, too! [Katy laughs] I was like, 'What the hell, that is so cool! I want to do that!'

After that exercise I remember we had to talk to the person next to us. I talked to (a mutual trainee friend) and she was just so nice, so kind, so open. It was a bit of a shaky thing to have to do in front of a whole bunch of people that I didn't know; I didn't know what the response would be, because I hadn't had a lot of history of coming out to people by then. I had come out to some friends and family, but it was a bit of a mixed history and not universally positive. In that training group I felt safe enough. I think that's because I knew quite quickly that I wasn't alone, so it felt okay quickly.

Overall, it really was a very positive experience. I didn't have any negative experiences at all in the training group. I had a sense that there was enough acceptance all round. I never felt dismissed.

When I came to do my dissertation, it was about my experience of being a cis female trainee therapist with a masculine gender expression. Describing myself like that still doesn't make me feel quite right, but I don't even know how else to describe it. I had discovered bow ties and gone, 'Oh! That's me!' I don't know whether to call it masculine, exactly, because it doesn't really sit with that word for me.

Either way, my dissertation was about gender expression, and I discovered that, actually, my training institute was a really nice place to experiment. I'd try new ties and bow ties and accessories, and I'd feel dead nervous, and I'd rock up for a training day and, in that little cocoon, I could see what response I was getting, and go, 'This is okay, actually.' But then I noticed that when I would go out for lunch, I'd put my anorak on and zip it right up to the top, because being 'out there' wasn't safe. The outside world was not trustworthy, but the training group was trustworthy. That's a definite distinction I made in my dissertation. I called it 'backstage' – the training institute was like a backstage area where I could experiment before I went to the front of the stage and go, 'Ta-dah!'

Katy: My memory of you experimenting with ties and bow ties was that people were so excited about it! Was that your experience, too?

Viv: Oh, yeah, definitely. I had a lot of real positive feedback. Nobody ever went, 'What're you doing that for?' or anything, there was none of that at all. People were really excited, and there was a real sense of people seeing my congruence in terms of my presentation of self, and they liked it! If I was wearing both nail varnish and a bow tie, they got that, too. It felt supportive, encouraging. I felt I could probably try anything and it would be alright, even when it felt so edgy to me. That was very helpful. I suppose maybe I'd have a different view now because there's more transphobia in the world but, blimey, if I couldn't go into a group of person-centred therapists that I know and be able to experiment with something and not expect something positive back, the world would be a really sad place. It's got to be the safest place, surely? And it was, for me.

Katy: What does queer person-centred therapy mean to you?

Viv: I've not really thought about it in those terms. I bring myself to my therapy work so, to that extent, it's queer. You could say that the person-centred approach is innately queer, almost. You know, it's like, 'Fuck all the conventions. Who are you as a person? I'm going to try and meet you, as you are, as I am, here, now.'

Katy: Do you think your queerness affects how you practise as a therapist?

Viv: I think being queer gives me some insight into a lot of experiences as a therapist. I can get things that perhaps other people would struggle to get. At the same time, I also have to be really mindful that my queer experience will be nothing like anyone else's experience. That's true of all therapists, isn't it, but it's something to be mindful of when there's something shared and yet it's really different. I do think it probably helps my capacity to empathize.

I'm not out as a therapist, generally speaking. I have a sort of allusion to it on my website. If people want to, and are capable of reading into what I've said about myself, they'll know. If they see that my dissertation was on gender presentation and think that's interesting, and see that I do work with LGBTQ youth, they can figure it out. But if they're not going to go there, they're not even going to twig that part of who I am.

In my dissertation I wondered whether I would start wearing bow ties as a therapist. I have never done that. It wouldn't be right to me. It might be a bit disruptive of the space given that, actually, most of my clients are straight. It's not something I've ever experimented with.

Katy: This has me thinking about something that I remember from when we were in training. I remember that you asked your therapist at the time if they were LGBTQ+, and she left the question with you for a long time before she answered it.

Viv: I think that was because she was obviously feeling the elephant in the room, which was that there was some attraction. Certainly I was intrigued by her, and attracted in some ways. She was the one who brought that up and asked if I wanted to know – it was that way around. She named a thing that she was definitely feeling and that I was doing my best to ignore, because that seemed like the safest route to walk. So she named it and asked me whether I wanted to know or not, and that's what I took away to ponder. Do I or don't I, and what does it mean either way?

It's funny, because I think I'd been seeing her for at least a year. I picked her. I knew from the second I saw her that she was going to be the right therapist, and now she would say some of that was some sort of attraction, or recognition of the other. There was a fellow feeling of 'this looks like a good match' that happened straight away. I knew that she'd be a good therapist for me, and she was, which in itself is a bit baffling to me still. I had been doing my best for all of that not to be relevant – if it was attraction, then I had to ignore it. That meant there was a big part of me that was missing from that therapeutic relationship. I was doing my damnedest to ignore it, and she was obviously much more congruent.

I took about two weeks to think about it, then I said, 'I think I would like to know,' and she told me she was, and it was a genuine surprise to me. I had managed to block out the possibility so carefully that I was genuinely surprised when, honestly, there was no reason to be surprised. I felt like I didn't know what to do with that intensity – and, I mean, it's intense anytime, isn't it, the therapeutic space? There must have been something about keeping myself safe, defended, hidden. I was like, 'Oh my god, I can't talk about that. How on earth am I going to talk about feeling attracted to my therapist, *to* my therapist, who's sitting right in front of me?' It was definitely helpful to know and to talk about it. The elephant in the room disappeared. Well, it didn't disappear, but it wasn't an elephant any more.

Katy: It sounds so useful that this was something you could process together. Has anything like that ever happened the other way around?

Viv: I haven't had that experience in reverse with clients. I've only had a few lesbian adult clients, and sometimes it's felt like they were reading me in certain way, but I felt it wasn't something that needed exploring because we weren't exploring anything about their sexuality. I know some people are better at reading and assuming, which sometimes happens in the therapy room.

Katy: It sounds like, for you with your clients, your identities aren't stuffed away somewhere during therapy but they're not right at the centre.

Viv: There's never been a time when I felt it would have been appropriate to say, 'Wouldn't it be helpful to know my sexuality?' Because that's quite a big thing, isn't it? I think it's really introducing something personal when it's not about me. So, no, I've not explicitly come out to a client. I can think of one client who I would definitely say had figured it out. It was apparent, but it wasn't made explicit because it didn't need to be. There were just some then shared cultural references, and that was kind of enough. It was quite wholesome!

Katy: Before this interview we talked about the potential anxieties around doing this interview together. I know that you also do some specialist work with anxious clients. Is there a particular way that you work with anxiety and 'inner critic' issues?

Viv: In the last couple of years, what I've found really helpful has been thinking in terms of configurations of self. I find Janina Fisher's *Healing the Fragmented Selves of Trauma Survivors* really helpful, both the book itself and the general approach.

I've been working with aspects of self that feel like they have a way of being in the world – not in a way that feels like dissociation or splitting my self up, but in terms of parts. I know I have a youngish part who's probably about 10, and who actually seems to provide a lot of my personality, and is really interested in everything. She wants to know, 'What about this? How does that work? Why do you do that? What does that do? Where might you find a tortoise in the desert? What about a tarantula?' A lot of that interest is excitement about the world, but it's also kind of anxious, with the aim of preventing things from going wrong. So, together, we'll be dead organized, really thinking ahead and getting stuff sorted. She's named, and I can talk to her and I get her feelings back.

I noticed a couple of years ago, when I was working with some clients and the work was really challenging, I would be feeling so anxious beforehand. I'd find myself needing to research and write notes intensely before seeing these clients. I realized it was this younger part of myself, or those aspects of myself that I can imagine as belonging to that young part. I was swamped with her anxiety. What I started doing was just reassuring her that she doesn't have to come to these sessions. She can stay safe, because it's nothing to do with her, because I'm the one who's the adult. I'm the one that's trained as a therapist, so I'll do the session. My younger self doesn't have to be adultified any more. She can just go off and do whatever. It's made such a difference! It's a complete revelation. Suddenly I wasn't feeling that anxiety at all. It's like, of course I know what I'm doing! It was such a useful learning for me, and it's cool that you can then talk to that part and go, 'This isn't for you, though. It's all right. You don't have to do this.' It helps you to be really compassionate with yourself, really gentle and understanding. You can say to your younger anxious parts, 'Of course you're worried, because you don't know anything about this! But I do. It's not your job to worry.'

So parts work has been really helpful to me in terms of my own anxiety. I quite like doing that sort of parts work with clients, too, as it can be very helpful, both generally and particularly with anxious clients.

Katy: It's so interesting how our younger configurations can try to protect us.

Viv: It's so interesting to me that she wants to protect me by having everything written down. It's what I've done for this interview, actually, because I've got notes in front of me, haven't I?!

With parts work you can also run into inner critics, as you mentioned earlier. I would see every part as having a positive role, but that role might just not apply to the here and now any more. Having a critical part was probably much more helpful back then, when you had to behave in a particular way or watch what you said or what you did to avoid punishment. It helps to remember that your inner critic was there for a good reason, and so it helps to give that part just as much understanding and compassion. I've helped clients see that, too.

Katy: That's been part of my way of working with inner critics, too. How has that part helped you in the past? Can that part of you find a different way of helping?

My inner critic has always been so loud, so something else I've done is deliberately establish a 'cheerleader part' to kick my inner critic out of the passenger seat! Now I can prioritize listening to the part of me that's rooting for my comfort and success.

Viv: A cheerleader part – that seems great!

I know that some people are very connected with their different parts, and I also think that parts work can be really helpful even if you're not really noticing that there are other parts there. All of those experiences can be real. I know that my parts are real, and they feel very real to me. I have at least three, all of which cope with different difficulties or are processing very early attachment. I think at least holding that as a possibility is helpful, so you can wonder what is a part of your present that is connected to your past. Is what you're going through now all coming from 'present you', or does it feel familiar in some way, maybe from way back? Maybe you can introduce a bit of dialogue and see what happens?

Something that I've done with myself and clients, that's referenced in *Healing the Fragmented Selves of Trauma Survivors*, is an exercise to help any inner child configurations feel safe. Sometimes, when we have really adverse early experiences – and many LGBTQ people do – our childhood self tends to be more of a separate part of our selves as we become adults. Maybe that part isn't identified quite as such by the client, or maybe it's very apparent to the client, but either way this exercise can be helpful. If you try to connect with that part, and you ask that part to look around, it probably still sees where it used to live – where it grew up. That young part does not know that, actually, it lives in a totally different room now. Maybe it's a much nicer room now, or maybe it's a whole house! You can invite that part of you to look around and know that, wow, times have changed. You can bring it up to the present. For me, that was astonishing, to introduce my very real childhood self to my happy adult life.

Katy: What's happy about your adult life now?

Viv: I feel way more connected with myself than I used to. I feel connected to all of my configurations, all of my parts. I really feel like we're working together – and I use 'we' loosely, because I know I'm not a 'we' as some people are a 'we'. I love knowing all of my self, and it means that I have more of a sense of doing things that are right for me. Having that awareness of those parts of me and what their pulls to my past are, I can see what's going on with my present feelings. I feel congruent. I have such a strong sense of valuing and connection with younger parts, and we can work together to have the best life. I love that.

I also love my work as a therapist, but I quite like that it's not so busy at the moment! Since Christmas 2023, some of my private practice clients have decided to go down to monthly sessions. Money's tight for most of my clients right now. A couple of clients also finished their work with me, so I'm left with a lot more gaps, and once I got past the shock and the worry, I'm kind of lapping it up. It means I've got a free Wednesday morning and I can go for a swimming lesson if I want. I can keep going to my pottery classes. I can use that time for myself.

In private practice I used to feel that constant tug between doing more client work and feeling the stability of money coming in, and taking the time that I need for myself. Do I fill the gaps again? Or do I just take a moment to breathe? I'm doing more breathing at the moment.

Katy: That sounds good. For me, rationally I know that these things balance out, and I can look over the whole last couple of years and see that I'm doing okay in my private practice, but still, every time I have a few gaps, I panic. This basically happens to me every summer, and I always make it out the other side!

Viv: Yes! It's like, 'Oh god, my clients have left, what am I going to do?' That wave of panic. It's going to be okay, though! I'm really feeling super balanced between my work and my self-care right now, and that is absolutely crucial.

Katy: I always find that having lots of time for proper self-care means you do your best work.

Viv: Oh, yeah. I prioritize my self-care, and the things I do for that, and I love how aware I am of what my self-care needs are.

Katy: How else has your work as a therapist changed over the last few years?

Viv: I'm not seeing anybody face-to-face as a therapist at the moment. I see clients on Zoom or talk over the phone – it's about half and half. My work with the survivors charity is all over the phone. You know, I wouldn't have imagined that all came about because of

COVID. Everything was face-to-face up to that point. It amazes me how deep that work can be, even though you can't see the person.

I still love being a therapist. It can be the hardest work in the world, and it can leave me absolutely flattened. I have to work real hard at processing, letting go of whatever it is I'm left with. Sometimes that's really hard, dependent on the client's situation, but other times, being a therapist is just joyous. It's still an absolute shock to me that I get to do this wonderful job. I wouldn't change it at all. Not for a second.

Katy: I'm glad that you're here, where you're supposed to be.

Viv: I'm glad that I'm here, too, and that I get to figure out where the future goes. I get to decide how long I keep doing this. I do have doubts, sometimes, but I think lots of people will do even when they love their work. It's okay to ask yourself if something is still right for you – and, so far, it is.

Katy: I think it's also okay if that changes again. It's okay to move from something you love to something better.

Viv: Absolutely! Continuing to think about this will be about being really responsive to myself.

Katy: [Half-joking] Maybe you'll find yourself as a famous pottery artist?

Viv: [Viv laughs] I think that's unlikely! I do find myself wondering if I could do an art course. I don't think I need to pass a course to love making art, though. I can just really enjoy what I'm doing and make sure that it pleases me and brings me joy. I'll keep doing what I'm doing at the moment. I've got a real good balance at the moment.

Katy: Have you noticed anything in particular that's making your queer clients feel unbalanced right now?

Viv: I feel for young people who are struggling with social media in particular. It brings a new kind of toughness to growing up LGBTQ. Yes, they've got the positive role models I didn't see as a child, but then they also get access to constant abuse. It's such a lot. I don't know how I'd feel as a queer young person these days. I wouldn't like to choose between isolation and knowing nothing, and just being scared. That fear that was around when I was young largely persists to this day, actually – we have not quite shaken it. Social media can show the really toxic side of what people have to cope with, and then you have to find a way to discard it. You don't have to take their toxicity in. Of course abuse will affect you but, if you can find a way to know that what they're saying doesn't change that you are good and whole and resilient, you can start to cast what they say aside. It isn't true, and you can keep it at arm's length.

Katy's post-interview thoughts

Before my interview with Viv I hadn't been aware of Goffman's theory of social dramaturgy (Goffman, 1956) but, as a neuroqueer person, these ideas around developing masks are familiar to me. Viv's experience of using her therapy training as a 'backstage' area to try on different kinds of gender expression before taking them into the 'real world' was one I was glad to hear about and participate in as a member of her 'audience', and it's helped me to reflect on how this is something I often offer to my therapeutic clients, too. I know I'm often one of the first people to see my clients experimenting with different gender presentations and different ways of unmasking. If gender is a performance (Butler, 1990), I'm glad that the queer community and the queer therapeutic world can offer a place for a supportive dress rehearsal.

Talking to Viv also reminded me to be extra-kind to my inner parts, who are all deserving of care and respect, even – especially? – my embattled inner critic. Looking to the different parts of yourself, as well as to your whole self, can be a complicated effort but one that's well worth it. My inner cheerleader says hi!

If you'd like to know more

Healing the Fragmented Selves of Trauma Survivors: Overcoming Self-Alienation, by Janina Fisher, 2017. Viv recommends this book during the interview as a source of inspiration for her personal and professional therapeutic work.

Gender Trouble: Feminism and the Subversion of Identity, by Judith Butler, 1990. Viv talks in this interview about exploring her gender performance, and it would be remiss of me not to recommend Judith Butler's original take on gender as performance, and how that influences all aspects of oppression, power, body norms, sexuality, and more.

No Bad Parts: Healing Trauma & Restoring Wholeness with the Internal Family Systems Model, by Richard C. Schwartz, 2023. This is an accessible book about parts work and self-directed compassion by the creator of the Internal Family Systems model, with useful exercises to follow and tools to try out.

Inclusive Therapy Training with LJ Potter

An introduction to LJ

LJ is a white, queer, polyamorous, kinky, non-binary, UK-based, person-centred therapist who uses per extensive knowledge in therapy skills, teaching, and GSRD (gender, sex, and relationship diversity; Davies and Barker, 2015) experiences to ensure queer voices are heard on all sides of the therapy dynamic. LJ uses a mix of pronouns for itself so, as I write about it, you'll see me using a mixture of per/person, meow/meows, and it/its pronouns, as well as its name.

As Sage Stephanou and I covered in their chapter at the beginning of this book, Western paradigms of therapy centre allocishet expectations of being, and this is often reinforced even in well-meaning training institutions. While clients often bring up sex and relationships in therapy, there is often little to no training offered in relational styles such as polyamory, ethical non-monogamy, and kink dynamics. This lack of training and understanding can leave uninitiated therapists of all levels feeling, at best, lost and confused (Carrington and Sims, 2024) and, at worst, actively hostile towards clients exploring different relational styles in therapy (Berke, Maples-Keller, and Richards, 2016).

LJ has an illustrious history of leading therapy training across institutions in England. Meows training and advocacy endeavours to move past allocishet ways of doing therapy and towards a true therapeutic understanding of GSRD clients and therapists. LJ was a year ahead of me in my therapy training, and the only other out non-binary person I knew who was training at my institution. I was looking forward to gaining a deeper understanding of per training experience, of queer training experiences in general, and how this has influenced person's current life as a therapy trainer.

LJ's interview

LJ: My name is LJ. It's the bane of my life, as far as names go. 'LJ – how do you spell that?' LJ. 'Just the letters?' Yes, just the letters. 'That's an interesting one.' 'What's your real name?' 'What's it stand for?' 'You're really just called LJ?' Yes, I'm just called LJ!

As far as pronouns go, that is something of a revolving journey. When you write this up or talk about this, I feel happier with a smattering of lots of pronouns rather than just picking one. You can also just use my name and not use any pronouns. Those options feel okay, because there just isn't anywhere that really feels at home.

I started out using they/them but didn't really like it. Actually, when I first started thinking about pronouns, I wanted to move to it/its, but I wasn't prepared for the emotional labour it would take to deal with everybody else's reactions to my choice of pronoun. Interestingly, I leverage this to my advantage these days, because I went to they/them, and then I created a neopronoun for myself and added meow as a pronoun. Some people I know have used meow for me, I've seen it. And then, if you've read *Woman on the Edge of Time*...?

Katy: You recommended it to me a while ago and I still haven't read it! I will. (I've since read it, and I loved it.)

LJ: In part of the book, the characters use per – short for 'person' – as a pronoun, and so about 18 months ago I adopted that.

When I was telling people, 'By the way, I've changed my pronouns from they/them to per,' everyone was like, 'That's really complicated,' so I was saying, 'I was originally gonna move to it/its pronouns,' and suddenly everyone was like, 'Oh, per is really good!'

Katy: [sarcastically] Oh, that's fun!

LJ: [Both laughing] I mean, bless them, they meant well! Everybody was just worried about how they don't want to objectify me. 'It/its' pronouns don't feel objectifying to me, but you don't have to get over that bit of your processing, because I'm not asking you to use it.

I've noticed that, in the 18 months I've been using per, I was happy others were using per for me, and I almost never used per for myself. That felt a bit unfair, to be using one set of pronouns for myself and requiring everybody else to do the work. And most people do, to be honest – most people have absolutely done the work.

These days it's a little complicated. I'm starting a new job on Monday next week, and I am not choosing to use 'per' there. It feels really difficult, because I feel like no pronoun particularly works for me. I just don't want 'she' to be used, so I don't really care what people use as long as they don't use she. I also really don't want people to default to they/them just because they can't use she. When I talk about myself, I usually avoid using a pronoun at all, and I'll just use my name, but that's a really difficult thing to get into an email signature!

I'm about to become a principal lecturer. I will be overseeing several courses related to counselling. I don't know quite yet what the job involves there, but that will be four days a week, and then one day a week I'll be working in private practice.

Currently – in my private practice – I work wholly with queer people in some form or another. I don't restrict my practice to that, but those people are the people who find me.

So, yeah, that's who I am and what I do. I'm here. I'm still going. I love what I do. If my employers would just let me do my actual job and stop handing me so much paperwork, I'd love it even more!

Katy: Are there any parts of your work that you're particularly proud of?

LJ: I really love being part of therapy training. When I left my last university job I had so many students emailing me saying, 'You made this possible for me, especially neurodivergent students saying, 'I wouldn't have got through this without your understanding.' I put things in place, like standing at the front of the room at the start of the year and saying, 'You can stim. There is a box of stim toys here. It's coming around the room – please take whatever you want and keep it to stim with. If you need to move, move. If you're struggling with eye contact, I'm not ever going to tell you – and no one on this course is going to tell you – that you need to work on your eye contact. As long as you can demonstrate that you are being empathic with your clients, eye contact is never going to be a thing that comes up.'

Katy: That is so cool; so needed.

LJ: I help students talk to their clients about how they use stim toys as therapists, rather than telling them that they've got to sit still, and cross their hands, and not cross their legs. I guess the work I'm most proud of has been making the course more inclusive.

I've had a blind student this year and, in his goodbye email to me, he said, 'You helped me with accommodations for things I didn't know I needed.' I was able to understand his accommodations and take those into consistent account. I'm really glad to have done that.

I didn't do it alone – I had contact with another lecturer who also teaches a person-centred approach and who's blind, and so I had a chat with him about what might be helpful. I'm glad that I've been able to do this and make those accommodations, and put in place a course that tries really hard to be inclusive.

As far as I'm aware, we're the only course in the country that runs explicit, external, safer spaces for racially minoritized students. My only regret is that we don't run a similar thing for queer students or other students struggling with issues around structural inequality. We have a 'safer space group' for racially minoritized students, and it meets once a term or at least three times a year. It's not enough, but I know it's been really useful for students because they've told me so. As far as I'm aware, we're the only course in the country that attempts to do anything like that for racially minoritized students. It's not marketed in any way, because 'the powers that be' struggle to know how to market this in a way that doesn't say, 'We're really racist, and we need to give you a safe place to go because we're so racist, and you won't survive without it.' I'm glad that we do it, I'm just a bit sad that the wider message isn't out there and that we can't recruit more inclusively as a result of having it. Students find out about it at open day, but they don't find out about it before they apply to university.

On the queer front, just by virtue of being queer and standing up at the front of the room at the start of term, students feel safer to come out. I had two students come out as trans midway through the year last year.

I helped to organize TPCA's (The Person-Centred Association) person-centred gender and sexuality conference in 2023. I wasn't able to go, but one of my students went and, on my last day of term when I said goodbye to him, he said, 'I went to the encounter. There were all these trans students talking about what a hard time they were having on their course, and I couldn't connect with any of it.' That was so brilliant to hear!

I know that this is because of me, and it's not me. I know that the course wouldn't have thought about all this if I wasn't there, but it won't go away now that I've gone away. There's a whole wider atmosphere and ethos that's been created and leaves a legacy. I'm really glad to have been able to do this.

Katy: What a great legacy to leave behind. It sounds like there's already so much for you to be proud of.

LJ: People say that, but I think it's just part of being a decent human being, surely? And would I think about it as much if I didn't apply these demographics to myself?

I feel like being queer has forced me to do much more work around race. Students have told me that I do more than any other white lecturers that they've known, and that I've been the first white lecturer to bring up racism in therapeutic spaces. I'm not afraid to stand at the front of the room and talk about the white lens through which everybody sees me and through which I see the world – it just seems so bizarre to some people that I might want to acknowledge that fact. I think, probably, if I weren't queer, I would be a lot more worried about doing that. I just think that, obviously I'm struggling with these things as a queer person, and I'm white, and I have much more privilege there, so it brings me to trying to think about other ways of being, and what that's like. I'm not perfect and I make mistakes, but I'm happy to be challenged and learn.

Katy: What drew you to working as a person-centred therapist?

LJ: I can remember this really clearly. I was asked that question when I interviewed for my therapy training course, and what I said was that it's really easy for me to retreat to an expert position and hide behind techniques and skills. I didn't want to take the risk of becoming an expert in the therapy room, because that can set up some really black and white thinking in me – that I know better than you do, and you need to do this, and if you don't do this then you're failing. I didn't want to take the risk of being that therapist. Person-centred therapy is a way to be a therapist where the only thing I need to do is be me, and there are no particular 'tools' that are required. There's no 'thought record sheet' in a person-centred approach – instead, there's empathy. If I can't do empathy, then I can't be a person-centred therapist, and that's the only thing that I think I really need. Being empathetic is what gives me a good read on a situation that I'm in, and I wanted something that centred that experience, rather than being able to retreat to some kind of expert safety.

I specifically chose a training institute that could do person-centred training. I know how to talk. I didn't need to learn how to talk. I needed to learn how to listen. Person-centred seemed to be the way to do that, rather than anything like CBT. I mean, the best CBT isn't just about pushing sheets at people, but CBT in the UK under the National Health Service is not the best CBT. I do know a CBT private therapist who works for two years or more with clients and probably does it in a much more humanistic, person-centred way, but that's rare. I didn't want to be that kind of integrative therapist that will just whip out a worksheet when they're stuck for what to do – and I know that's not what it's supposed to be, but at its worst, that's what it is. Maybe I'm a bit of a snob, as well – I wanted me to make the difference, rather than any tools! [Both laugh]

I don't know. Sometimes, I think about all the things that I thought I knew when I applied for my training that I didn't know at all. Some of what I thought was important is very different now.

Katy: That has me thinking back to my own training interview and cringing a bit! So, yeah, I get that!

LJ: Yeah! There was just something about the training institute I trained at. I remember walking in there for the first time and not having a clue where I was going. I remember getting there and being met downstairs. We went right up to the top of the building for the interview, into one of the smallest rooms. I remember, I walked in the front door and went, 'This is where I want to be.' In that moment, I walked in and it felt like home.

Katy: I'm so glad that you got to have that experience.

LJ: I mean, at that point, yes. It started well. It was downhill from there.

Katy: What was it like for you to be a queer therapist in training?

LJ: It was hard. As you know, I don't have an MSc, I just have a PGDip (a postgraduate diploma) because being queer in training felt too difficult. It's necessitated some interesting conversations with the institute over time.

I was so angry in training. I constantly felt like I was being missed. We had a lecture on attachment and, all the way through, the lecture slides talked about the mother. I said, 'Where's the father? Or, you know, the other mother, but like, where's the father's responsibility in all of this?' And one of the trainees on my course said to me, 'Well, that's just implied.'

Katy: How ridiculous!

LJ: I felt like I was the only person doing this work. I transitioned in the start of my second year there. It's not all about gender and sexuality – some of it's just about me – but I felt like an outsider all the time there, and that made me so angry all of the time. I was too angry to be properly reflexive. Because I was so angry, I couldn't see past it a lot – there was a lot for me to have learned in all of that and I couldn't learn it.

I still feel hard done by, to be fair, because I don't feel like I was facilitated. I just kept being asked, 'Have you taken this to therapy?' I had, but that wasn't the issue – this was a structural problem that they were making my personal problem. Nobody would take enough of a risk to help me.

Other students faced difficulties, too. There were two people in my cohort who were Black. It was seven at one point, and became two over time. I was talking to one of them recently; I messaged her and said, 'I'm really sorry. It never occurred to me to think intersectionally about any of this stuff, and we certainly didn't learn about racism on the course. I never considered your experience as a Black woman.' She said 'I never thought about it while I was on the course, either.' She talked to me about her life post-qualification. She lives in a small town and she was saying to me, 'I don't know whether to put my photo next to my name. What does it do if don't have a photo, and what does it do if I'm a visibly Black woman?' I'm really sorry that I never took her intersections into consideration during training. I don't think anyone else did, either. I was so angry about my own mistreatment all the time, and I felt so unsupported, and it just felt like everything was being hushed up.

Now I know more about the culture of what was happening there at the time. I'm also given to believe that my experience was a catalyst for change. I certainly do know that trans students studying there now are having good experiences. I spoke to someone maybe 18 months ago online, and their they/them pronouns popped up on screen, and they said they were studying at this training institute, so I pinged them a message to see how they were finding it, and they said it was really good and they were really supported in being trans.

Katy: What a relief!

LJ: So I know that things have changed but, at the time, I was just left with how awful it was. I don't regret going, but I don't think I could have stayed.

I also feel angry that I don't have my MSc – I definitely felt cheated. Grades mattered so much to me at the time. I'd just done an MSc and I got a distinction, so I was determined that I was going to get a distinction in this one, too. To have to think about leaving without even getting an MSc just felt like the end of the world to me. That taught me something about myself and where I placed my worth – I was able to go from needing to get a good degree to just needing to look after myself. I had two choices: my mental health, or my qualification. I feel glad that the qualification hasn't really mattered in my life, but I still feel angry about it sometimes.

Katy: Hearing you talk about this makes me wish I had done things differently. I remember reaching a similar stage – because of what felt like discrimination in training, and the financial cost, and other life things – and I chose the qualification over my mental health. I felt like I had to get to the end, because if I didn't have the MSc I wouldn't have a career. Ironically, clients almost never ask to see my qualifications.

LJ: I am glad that I left when I did but angry that I felt like I had to.

Katy: That makes me angry as well.

LJ: Equally, I feel angry knowing that I'm not the only person that's had that experience. Of course, I didn't think I was, but to hear it out loud is difficult.

I remember, in my last but one weekend of studying there, some-body in the group was talking about me, and he said 'they' for the first time, and then he was like, 'Yes! I got it right!' With a fist pump!

Katy: [Laughing in disbelief at this guy's audacity] Oh, god. Binary people, right?

LJ: Yes! I just couldn't do it anymore. I'm still in contact with a couple of people that I trained with, so it hasn't been all bad as an experience, but I do know there are things that I do really differently on my course as a result of those experiences and who I am. I feel sad at times – but also glad! – when I look at my trans students and I know what a decent experience they're having. I feel really sad that that couldn't have been my experience. I'm glad that other students are having a much better time. I do also absolutely respect that I have the freedom to do that in my courses that potentially wasn't around at the point when I was training.

Katy: I wish that we'd had the kind of time that your students have been having. What is it like now, to be on the other side and to be a queer therapy trainer and teacher?

LJ: Being a trainer is interesting. I mean, you talk about being a queer therapist. My sexuality never comes into it. When anybody wants to talk about me, they're not talking about my sexuality – it's the being trans thing that matters to everybody. When I train counselling students, their lectures are three and a half hours long. The first half is focused on LGBT, and the second half is poly and kink. Then they have a vignette case study to look at. Invariably the questions that we have at the end are about trans people. They're only asking questions about gender critical beliefs or being trans.

It's the same whenever I've done training with qualified therapists, too. I did a presentation on National Counsellors Day in 2022, and I presented on conversion therapy, and at least one person in the room was anti-trans but so insidious about it. I think the other people who were trans or queer in the chat were shutting it down, but the team managing it weren't doing anything. That person misgendered me several times, and they were corrected by people several times, and they kept going. So, if you're running a talk or a training session, you need to know that there are going to be these people. You will need people on your moderating team who know how to deal with this. It's something I'm more careful about now.

Still, I love doing the work and being a trainer. My students do some lectures about gender and sexuality at the end of term one. I always stand at the front of the room, with a whole slide that lists me as white, disabled, poly, kinky, trans, ace, and aro. I then talk about it all, and I talk about why I talk about it. If I want my students to be able to talk to clients without shame, then I can't do it without positioning myself in relation to that. I know that when I was training, for example, there was a session on kink, but it was an elective in the fourth year, so I never got to have it. I don't do lots with my students on kink, but learning some of the language is so important. If a client comes in and says something really basic – like, that they're a sub – then I don't want these therapists to be hearing that for the first time and going, 'What does it mean to be submissive?'

Katy: I get so many clients who are coming to me after having therapists like that!

LJ: There's also the pathologization. For example, I've had more than one client come because they've been given something like a BPD (borderline personality disorder) diagnosis, in part because they were polyamorous, bi, and/or kinky, because 'polyamorous people can't make commitments and bisexual people are indecisive'. I'm sorry, but if you think that then you've never seen the life of a poly person! We are committed! It's fucking difficult to be poly and not be committed to this!

Katy: It takes so much work to do it well!

LJ: Right! I've had those clients as well, that have been pathologized. Just because a psychiatrist knew they were bi and poly, to them that automatically meant they had BPD.

Katy: Sadly, I've heard of things like that happening so many times before from clients and people in my community.

LJ: Sometimes it feels absolutely terrifying to be doing this, to be standing up for these clients. I worry I'm going to be reported or doxxed for being trans and trans-positive. Sometimes it feels really terrifying to be a queer therapist and trainer who is so visible. It is terrifying to think that somebody could report me to my registering body on the grounds of promoting an ideology to students. I've had supportive teams and supportive students so far, but I'm very aware of how vulnerable I am.

Katy: I get that. Even if you know you're probably going to be safe, it's so difficult to not have that certainty, and to know that safety can change at any point.

LJ: When I talked to someone at the university about what we would do if a gender critical student wanted to make a complaint about me, she said, 'But why would they do that?' Because they don't believe that I am fit to be running a course, because they believe that I am delusional. 'Well, that's just ridiculous.' Yes, but it's not going to stop them from doing it. 'But why would they do something so unpleasant?' Because the unpleasantness is the point. She just couldn't understand it, that someone might do this.

Katy: What is it like now, to be a queer therapist?

LJ: I love being a queer therapist! I love knowing where my queer clients are coming from. I love when a client will say something about their queerness and I get to think, 'I know this, too.' That's important to pick up on and I will feed it back to my queer clients, that they're heard and understood.

Katy: What inspired you to work with an LGBTQ+, kinky, polyam client group?

LJ: This is something that, again, I remember really clearly. When I was training, I didn't really have a lot of options for placements, and certainly not while I was also working full time; all the placements wanted you to come during the day. I initially set up my counselling placement within a switchboard charity. They were reliant on funding, so they were always coming to us and saying, 'This is your three months' notice. If we don't get any funding in the next couple of weeks, then you've got only three months,' and this happened over and over. We didn't ever tell clients that we thought there might only be three months left, but we were just always on the brink of having to close next week. I decided I had to move the counselling placement to be a standalone service.

I added another counselling placement because I wasn't getting many hours. It was a sexual abuse centre. I told them I was non-binary and transitioning. They said it was fine, but the inflexion was that it was fine as long as I looked like a woman, sounded like a woman, didn't try to push my pronouns on anyone, and dressed the part.

Katy: Unfortunately, that doesn't surprise me.

LJ: No, nor me. I didn't last very long in that placement. I saw two clients who both had six weeks of sessions, so I lasted maybe two months in that service before I left, because of the ethos that was like, 'Yes, of course you can be here, as long as you don't actually do anything to tell anybody else who you are.'

I'm so glad that I had the privilege of being able to set up my own placement. After about nine months I took on someone else who was just qualifying, so we ran it between us, working to set up a charity. I chose to work with this client group because I wanted people to have a place where they could go where gender and sexuality could be explored without judgement. I wanted my clients to have a space where there was no risk of abuse or harassment because of who they are. I wanted clients to go somewhere where they could do that safe exploratory work.

I remember that somebody who was training with me asked me, 'Why do you only want to work with those people and those issues?' I was like, 'Which people? Because they're just people!' I really just want for people to be able to come into counselling and just be their queer selves. I want the therapists they see to know enough to talk about it but not to make it the issue.

For example, I might have a client who is a lesbian, but we're not really talking *about* her sexuality, it's just there. So, that client might not talk about struggling with outright homophobia but, if that client is talking about how stressed she's feeling, I might say, 'And, of course, there's all the additional stress of being a lesbian.' Clients tend to respond with things like, 'Yeah, you're right.' They might not have thought about it until that moment, but I might be really feeling it, and I don't think a straight therapist would have picked up on that. I know that minority stress is going to influence that experience, so I just want to make sure that clients specifically know that they are seen, and heard, and understood.

When I created the charity, I specifically wanted to create a place where people could come and be queer, and talk about whatever they wanted to talk about. In private practice, I've kept that going. The only place I list myself is on the Pink Therapy Directory. I'm guessing that 99% of people that come through there are queer, or think they might be, so that's where I've stayed.

Katy: What kind of topics do GSRD (gender, sex and relationship diversity) clients tend to bring to your private practice?

LJ: When I'm working with queer clients, the topics that I work with are all the topics. We're not limited to gender or sexuality. It's rare that people want to come and talk about their sexuality or their gender as the main topic of conversation.

Katy: I find that, too. I have clients who want to come and figure things out, which is extremely welcome, but a lot of my clients are just looking for somewhere they can be queer in peace and talk about what's actually going on in their lives. Their queerness needs to be understood even if it's not at the centre of the discussion.

LJ: Absolutely. It's so often in the flavour of life. For example, if I have a client whose mother always misgenders them, that's the kind of thing I'm holding in mind when that client visits home, as well as everything else that might be going on with travelling to see family. They might not say anything about it, or anything else about their visit home, but it's important that they know that I know that they had that experience, whether or not they choose to talk about it this time.

Katy: That's such a needed knowledge for queer folk. Do you find that's similar for kinky clients, and clients in the BDSM community, too?

LJ: Most of the time, I find kinky clients just want to bring 'life stuff', and the kink stuff is incidental.

When kink comes up, it's often about working through preferences, navigating boundaries, and making discoveries about themselves. Sometimes it's about finding something they like that's surprised them, or about finding hard limits, or wondering if they can work through a limit.

It's also quite often about the logistics. It's situations like, 'I really love this person, but we're both sub-leaning switches. How do we make this work in a way that feels okay?' It's the kind of conversation you'd have about vanilla relationships – it could be any small incompatibility, it just happens to be about kink.

Sometimes I do have clients talking about kink and looking for reassurance that they're not wrong for being that way. They sometimes ask for reassurance that they're not bad for being kinky in some way, and that they're not broken.

I don't tend to see very much BDSM-related soul-searching, especially with LGBTQ+ clients. I think that's died down with the advent of *Fifty Shades of Grey*, much as I absolutely loathe it! That series is partly why I teach kink dynamics so early – therapists need to be able to tell the difference between coercion and a D/s (Dominant/ submissive) dynamic, and ask the right questions when they're not sure.

I've definitely had clients come to me and say things like, 'So I went to stay with one of my partners this weekend,' and then ten minutes later they've gone, 'Your profile said you're kinky...' I'm always like, 'Yes, I am,' and I prepare myself a little. Then they say, 'So, anyway, that partner was my Daddy,' and that changes everything completely! When clients bring things like this, I think it's often because they wanted to test out my understanding.

So, by and large, kinky clients come to talk about non-kinky things, but they've sought out a kink-knowledgeable therapist because they want to know that kink can be something they reference that I won't pathologize them for.

Katy: Do you find it's the same with polyamorous clients, too?

LJ: It can get really complicated when you're working through relationship dynamics that are like, this is your triad here and this is your quad here, but at least one person out of your triad is also in your quad, and I have to hold all of that and remember everyone! But clients aren't usually talking to me about how that's a struggle.

Katy: What are the main differences you see between polyamorous and monogamous clients?

LJ: I think the main differences that I see are around intentionality. I think my clients get that intentionality from me, too, as a polyamorous therapist, because I am challenging those default assumptions.

I tend to find that monogamous clients have sets of default assumptions that polyamorous clients don't tend to have. I also find that polyamorous clients are far more likely to prioritize talking to their partners to solve problems. The working assumption for many polyamorous people is that, in order to be poly successfully, you have to communicate – I don't find that for monogamous clients, oddly. You just have to move in together and your job is done! That's you for the next 20 years, until something goes wildly wrong! [Both laugh]

I'm generalizing here, of course. Many monogamous people absolutely believe in prioritizing communication to resolve problems, and lots of polyamorous people do not. But that is a big one, that poly clients tend to be more forward and deliberate in their intentions. By and large, I find that my poly clients are more prepared to have the difficult conversations with their partners without having to come to therapy to think about those hard conversations, whereas monogamous people will come and they'll want to talk through something about their relationship, their connection, before they talk to the other person. Polyamorous clients tend to come to session and be like, 'This thing happened, so we've organized a round table conversation and I've set up a meeting with my metamour' (a partner's partner). They'll put communication into action and come to therapy to process after the fact, whereas monogamous clients tend to want to process things before, during, and after.

So there's something about proactiveness for polyamorous

people. Maybe we can't afford to assume that everything will be fine if we don't talk about it? I remember before I became polyamorous, when I was dating my girlfriend. She kissed someone else, and I was talking about this online to someone I met, and telling them about how she cheated on me. The person said, 'Did you have a conversation about whether or not you were going to be monogamous?' And we had not. Whereas, in all my relationships now – and I see poly clients doing the same thing – we'll be talking all of this through.

Another difference I see is in talking about STI (sexually transmitted infection) testing with partners very openly. The amount of lesbian women – and others – who have no clue what their STI status is, is just out there. Almost everyone I know who's polyamorous knows exactly what their status is and when they were last tested. There's a lot more concern for physical well-being and wanting to make sure that their partners are aware of where they are in that process. I guess it comes back to that relational intentionality.

Katy: Is there anything you would like to tell queer, kinky, and polyam people who might be looking for therapy?

LJ: Find out what your potential therapists know. Don't put up with a therapist who is going to need a 101, or pretend they know what they're talking about.

About three years ago I was reading a post on Facebook, and a counsellor there said, 'My client was telling me all about being trans today and I didn't understand it, so I was asking them all sorts of questions, but it's okay because I didn't charge them.'

Katy: There's a lot going on there.

LJ: Yeah. I have current trans student therapists, who have had their therapy turned into 'tell me what it's like to be trans' sessions. As trans and queer people it's all too easy to feel grateful. We can feel too grateful when someone knows what a label means or remembers our pronouns – and I've been there, I've done that.

So find a therapist who, on first impression, doesn't leave you thinking, 'I'll take this one because they've not been openly hostile.' You can interview your therapist and find out what your therapist thinks about gender and sexuality and how those things play into our daily lives. It's okay to ask them, 'Are you really okay with polyamory in all of its forms? Are you really okay with kink?' It's okay to work with a therapist who doesn't know much about these things, as well, but be aware of what your therapist thinks about these identities.

On the other side of things, there are therapists who won't even want to deal with your queerness at all. They should also be avoided. When I was training and I needed my 40 hours of personal therapy, there were only two therapists in my area who fitted the training institute's criteria. Long story short, I fired both of them and eventually was allowed to go back and see my good original therapist who didn't quite meet the criteria. But, in my search, I rang up a counselling centre and said, 'I'm doing counselling training. I'm required to be in weekly therapy as part of my training.' They said this was no problem. I said, 'So, I'm poly. I'm kinky. I'm trans. These are not things that I am bringing to therapy particularly – I'm fine with all of those identities – I just need to be in therapy.' And they said, 'Oh no, you're too complicated for us.'

Katy: Oh, for god's sake!

LJ: I know, it's just ridiculous, isn't it?

When I teach, I teach a vignette about a client called Charlie. Charlie is 23, is a polyamorous submissive, and is wondering if a current partnership is the right type of connection for them. Their partner isn't named, but he's a decade older. I then have a whole list of questions about things like, 'What don't you know in this situation? When might you refer on? What concerns do you have? How would these concerns be different, depending on how you're gendering this client? How would those concerns be different depending on the client's age?' My clients almost always assume – decide – that Charlie is a woman. Nobody decides that Charlie is non-binary. They always decide that Charlie is a young woman and that, because she is dating a kinky man who is 10 years older than her, she is being groomed. I get the students to talk about what it would be like if Charlie was a 23-year-old man, for example.

All this is to say you need a knowledgeable therapist who you know is interrogating their assumptions. Rather than just taking the first therapist who doesn't screw up, we can take the time to interview therapists and say, 'What's your experience? What's your understanding? What makes you think you're a good fit for me?' If you're gonna go to therapy, write some questions down. Check out pinktherapy.com and ask the therapists you find there some questions. Otherwise, I think we are in danger of accepting subpar therapy.

Katy: How do you think the therapy profession is changing for queer therapists right now?

LJ: I do think things are changing. Have you heard about the Pink Therapy mentoring scheme that I started for Dominic (Dominic Davies, the founder and CEO of the organization Pink Therapy)?

Katy: Yes! I didn't know you started that! That's amazing!

LJ: It's a great scheme. The thing is, they always have loads of cis gay men who want to help, but they don't have loads of cis gay trainees who want help. They have lots of non-binary trainees and not so many non-binary therapists out there with spoons. (By 'spoons', LJ is referencing Spoon Theory, a metaphor for how chronically ill and disabled people may have limited energy levels, or fewer 'spoons' than others.)

But the political climate is changing. Things are getting better, and also things are getting worse. I think that our identities will become much more politicized in the counselling arena, and we are in for a difficult time.

Katy: I can see that starting to happen, unfortunately.

LJ: I'm glad that we have things like the mentoring scheme, and groups like TACTT (Therapists Against Conversion Therapy and Transphobia). TACTT do some really good stuff, and I am part of the administration team. They recently wrote and organized an open letter to UKCP (UK Council for Psychotherapy) about their decision to withdraw from the Memorandum of Understanding to ban conversion therapy. I didn't have a hand in writing it, but it was a good letter.

Katy: It was a great letter. I was proud to sign it.

LJ: I'm not sure it will make a difference.

Katy: I am trying to be optimistic about that.

LJ: We already have students citing the recent UKCP statement on conversion therapy that promoted TACTT's open letter. We have students citing that letter as evidence as to why they should be allowed to carry out conversion therapy. I think the counselling field is going to get a lot more complex for trans topics, and for trans therapists, before it gets better. I have hope that it will come around eventually, but right now I think it's gonna get harder before it gets easier. I think we are in need of more networking and more kinds of support.

I want to see queer therapy go to some really lovely places, and I think it could, but first we have to get through all of the gender critical stuff. Every time I hear about it, I just feel worse and worse.

At least I can make sure my students have a decent understanding of trans and queer topics, because I'm trans and queer at the front of the room every week.

Katy's post-interview thoughts

I came away from LJ's interview with a real felt-sense of what a gift it is to be a GSRD therapist for my GSRD clients. It doesn't always feel like a gift; it certainly didn't feel that way during my training, where I made wonderful queer friends but also felt completely missed in so many ways. Like LJ, I had some similarly transphobic and queer-phobic run-ins during my therapy training and placements, as well as facing down microaggressions borne of classism, ableism, and fatphobia. I also saw the number of trainees of colour in my training group dwindle drastically over time, expressing that they did not feel welcome in the training environment, which I'm still grieving. My therapy training was one of the best things I have ever done – in a lot of ways, it made me who I am, and I quite like who I am – but, also, the way training has traditionally been conducted has actively kept marginalized therapists from progressing through training, and kept marginalized clients from accessing good therapy.

I am so glad to hear that this is changing. It's been a pleasure and a relief to hear that my therapeutic alma mater has stepped up towards anti-oppressive therapy training, and that trainers like LJ are out there doing the work to make sure queer therapists and clients are all cared for.

If you'd like to know more

Pink Therapy Directory. LJ mentioned this as a resource for finding LGBTQ+ knowledgeable therapists. The Pink Therapy Directory is an online directory of trusted therapists and counsellors who are committed to working with GSRD clients. You can search for a mental health professional in your area and/or online, and you can make specific searches depending on the type of care you need and the GSRD identity of potential therapists. https://pinktherapy.com/find-a-therapist

Pink Therapy mentoring scheme. LJ helped to start this mentoring scheme for therapists and counsellors. The aim of the scheme is to link trainee therapists with established therapists who share aspects of queerness in common, with the hope of growing connections and experiential knowledge within the LGBTQ+ therapy profession. https://pinktherapy.org/mentoring

Therapists Against Conversion Therapy and Transphobia (TACTT). TACTT is a lobbying group of therapists who are committed to fighting conversion therapy and transphobia in the mental health profession and beyond. LJ is part of TACTT's organizing committee. https://therapistsagainsttransphobia.org

Woman on the Edge of Time, by Marge Piercy, 1976. LJ's use of per/person pronouns came about after reading this book, where characters living in a utopian future society use these gender neutral pronouns. I've since read this book and loved it for its takes on transformational madness and neuroqueerness as a part of paradise.

The Forensic Psychiatric System with Rory

An introduction to Rory

Rory (she/they) is a mental health worker, anti-sex-trafficking advocate, and forensic psychology student from the UK. On TikTok, as *dxgitalfootprxnt*, their content explores their life as a queer, Black, neurodivergent, disabled person living within the psychiatric care system, as well as their life as a master's student, feminist, and hamster parent.

I've known Rory for about ten years – or, more accurately, I've known Rory's system for about ten years. Rory was not the host of her system when we first connected in a Facebook group about toxic masculinity. I've connected with several of the other people in their system, all of whom have been incredible in their own way. Rory herself has been a fierce and delightful friend to me for several years.

Rory's system is currently safely living in supported housing while studying to work in forensic psychology. At the time of this interview, they were residing in a rehabilitation unit. She has been living under some kind of psychiatric care for most of the time I have known her, and she has been working hard to help others for even longer. Seeing the work she's done for herself and for others has been a delight, and seeing how she has been treated by the mental health systems she should have been able to rely on has been unbearable to watch.

Including people like Rory, LGBTQ+ people have a long history of being detained (Villarreal, 2023), medicalized (Ford, 2013; Burton, 2024), and criminalized (Panfil, 2018). While LGBTQ+ people face higher levels of trauma and are more likely to need psychiatric help (Berke *et al.*, 2016; Hatzenbuehler *et al.*, 2024), especially when combined with other aspects of discrimination like racism (Van-Bronkhorst *et al.*, 2021), much that happens in the current carceral and psychiatric systems does not adequately care for LGBTQ+ detainees. The effects of this can be felt from acute mental health settings (Fadus, Hung, and Casoy, 2020) to long-term forensic settings (Gorden *et al.*, 2017). The main components that tend to make mental health care ethical and effective, like client agency and mutual trust, are so often missing from these settings (Wren, 2021) and are deliberately omitted from carceral systems.

Luckily, there are people like Rory who are determined to set things right.

Rory's interview

Rory: I am Aurora, but everyone calls me Rory. That is not our body's legal name; I am in a DID (Dissociative Identity Disorder) system.

I'm 31, and my pronouns are she/they. I don't really mind which one is used. I don't think any of my others really mind that much, because the ones that do mind about their own pronouns would probably understand that this is fine for me.

I'm also in a relationship with my fiancée, who is an angel. She proposed to me at the beginning of January 2024. She is very supportive and has been there for me over what's been probably the roughest years of my life whilst I'm residing where I live.

I'm a forensic psychology student. That, honestly, is difficult, but it will be worth it. While it's hard, I need to do it because I think that's going to be beneficial in my future no matter where I want to go with that.

I currently live in an open rehabilitation place after living in secure for a really long time, and doing my treatment for lots of years. I started my degree whilst in a secure setting, which was probably what made it really difficult to start with.

Katy: What drew you to study forensic psychology?

Rory: I've always worked in settings where I've been caring for others. My first real job was as a youth worker, after I'd been working voluntarily as a youth worker when I was under the age of 18. I worked with over-25-year-olds who were young mums. My own youth worker at the time was like, 'You need to come and do this because if you're not going to go to school, you're doing this. It's here to help you.' And it did! I really enjoyed it, so then I was officially offered the job.

When I hit 18 I got offered a role to be a PAYP worker (Positive Activities for Young People). I had my own caseload; it's a lot more intense. I didn't really know that at the time, but I was like, [playfully unconvinced] 'I'll do the training...!' [Rory laughs] But I did really enjoy it. I know my own lived experiences helped. That was when I realized that I want to be able to help people that not only have issues that they need guidance with, but also that are little bit more complex, where they need support workers with lived experiences and good training.

Even when I got quite poorly, I still did my work from home and hospitals. I made sure that I kept up to date with my emails and any groups that I needed to do online, until my boss was like, 'You need to look after yourself!' I needed to do a lot of self-preservation with that, and manage my system, so that everyone in my system understood that need to look after ourselves. At that time I wasn't fully hosting, so I was just like, 'Hello? Are we listening to me? Is anybody listening to me?' It was difficult for me, because I was used to micromanaging and mass-managing everything, and then I wasn't any more. I still tried to be around a lot, just to make sure that we – as a whole – could get to where we needed to be, to be able to help people back at a healthier level where we weren't exhausting ourselves.

Then, we ended up going into hospital to stay. We started doing our psychology degree, and we got that okay. I wasn't too fussed about passing that, but I think that's probably because I wasn't the one doing it! So I was just like, 'Hmmm, this is anticlimactic!' But, while I was in hospital, I was noticing around me that there isn't really much care for the younger people, or the older people, or those that are quite severely ill. It felt like it was such a small circle of people in the mental health system that could get proper care. Instead, it tended to be that you'd go into hospital, your meds would change, and you'd leave, but then you ended up coming back, and then it just spiralled further. I didn't like that.

So, further on in time, when I'd gone through different secure units and different mental health situations, I thought, 'I want to do forensics because there's people that are missing out.' That's why I started my forensic psychology studies.

It reminded me of when we were first volunteering – when I was around a little bit more, when we were younger – and we worked with the young mums. I remember we were looking into what support the prison service offers to mothers that don't have access to their kids while they're in prison, and there isn't much at all. It's another bad pattern – they'd go to Mother and Baby Units; they're not looked after; they don't get given the correct support; their kids are taken; and then they're just told to carry on for the rest of their time in prison. I want to help fix that. I want to be able to build something in that area. That's the main thing that I want to do. I've seen so much in my own personal life that I want to make a difference somehow, even if it's one small difference. That's one difference more than nothing.

Katy: This sounds like it's going to make a lot of difference. The work that you've already done has made a lot of difference, too. I really hear you on how important this is – these people are so often missed.

Rory: Definitely, which is sad. I want it to be thought about more, because I don't think people do think about it. Everybody that I've spoken to about it – even at university – when I've explained and told them what I want to work towards, they've been like, 'We don't really hear that very often. Forensic psychologists usually want to work at hospitals and we thought that, because you've had a lot of hospital experience, you'd want to work there.' That's something I could do, but my main aim is to help those that are marginalized in the prison system, and the youth that have been in the prison system, because they get shut down a lot.

Yes, okay, they may have broken laws. Everybody's broken a law. I don't care – rules are rules, laws are laws, and that doesn't mean that, if you're unwell, you don't deserve to have something to make you feel well. It doesn't matter how you got to where you are.

Katy: Absolutely, I totally agree. What has studying forensic psychology been like for you so far?

Rory: Studying has actually been so positive for me. There are so many different options. I study forensic psychology with the Open University (OU), which has been so good as somebody that's neurodivergent. I can't just go and study someplace physically – no, thank you, I'm not doing that! [Both laugh] I've been given so many different resources. There are different types of groups and virtual online meet-ups, and different lectures, and different tutorials.

I've also got a support worker through my Disabled Students Allowance. That was difficult to deal with at the beginning because I was overwhelmed. I was sorting that and student finance all at the same time. But then I realized I can just say, 'I don't know what I'm doing; help me.' And they just do! They provided me with the things that I needed to be able to concentrate properly. They sorted my university laptop out for me, installed all of my speech-to-text stuff; they installed everything that I'd need. They even sorted out my ring binder booklets so I didn't have to continuously keep the page up, because I have a wrist problem.

So that scheme, and the OU, they're just very inclusive and they do the best they can. I genuinely have nothing but good experiences.

Katy: What is it like to be part of a neurodivergent plural system while working in mental health?

Rory: It's a complicated one. For me, I think I got very lucky. However, I look back on things and there were some times where the only reason I got lucky is because I already knew my supervisors, my managers, and my bosses from being a young person.

Working in mental health was difficult for me because, at the time, I'd just been diagnosed as autistic. There were certain things around me that were in place to make sure I could concentrate properly and do what I needed to, that were immediately put in place by my manager and my supervisor. Everyone above me did everything good for me, but it was the people that I worked with 'on the floor' that would pass judgement. It made me uncomfortable. I'm not great at standing up for myself in a professional way. In general, if somebody says something, I'll be like, 'What is wrong with you? Stop!' At work I'd find it really difficult because, if you're undermining me, and I'm trying to keep everything maintained on my level whilst giving you the respect that you deserve, I don't know what I'm supposed to say, so I'll just sit and I'll take it.

I also know that, when I got to the point where I had my own team and I was supervising, I still looked quite young and I got into the job role quite young. There was a point where someone new joined and it was difficult, because they spoke down to me all the time, even around the young people we were working with. Even when it came down to things like having to sign their timesheets, they were like, 'Why do I need to get you to sign it? I'll get my manager to sign it.' And I'd have to be like, 'I'm your supervisor. I can sign it. No big deal.' She'd make comments about my age and about certain aspects of our mental health that really didn't need to be said at all. 'I'm older than her. She looks poorly. She's underweight.' They didn't need to say any of those things. I was lucky, because I had the backup of my manager and my boss, and they were able to sit down and tell them that's not an acceptable way to treat your supervisor. This person didn't last in the job very long.

There were even times where I felt like I needed to walk out, because I didn't know how I could handle the situations with staff without crying. They'd be judging me out loud with our other colleagues that were also working under my team. It felt really lonely. In some ways it didn't help that I had a good relationship with management – my colleagues also began judging me because they knew I could go to the manager and the boss – they'd be like, 'You're gonna go run to the manager and the boss on us?' Which meant I then sometimes felt like I couldn't get help at all. I felt like I was being isolated; I felt very stuck. It was very uncomfortable.

I was lucky that I could go to somebody and say, 'This is what's happening. It's making me uncomfortable. I don't know how to handle the situation,' and they would guide me. How they taught me, they made sure they didn't just do it for me, but they'd also make sure that it was safe. I think, if I didn't have the people working above me that knew me really well and were good to me, it would have been really bad. It would have been hell. It would have really not been good for me.

I think there's positives and negatives in every situation. I cannot sit back and say it was all bad or all good. I can see that there's good and bad, but I personally know that I was likely luckier than most neurodivergent and mentally ill people, so I'm worried about the future. I won't always have that safety of somebody knowing and understanding what I need, but I think I've got enough skills to be able to assert myself professionally in settings, now. More than I did when I was a lot younger, at least.

Katy: It can be such a wild experience! I know a lot of wonderful colleagues and peers who work in mental health, but it always amazes me how often mental health workers are absolute bullshit about their colleagues' mental health stuff.

Rory: Right? It can be such a bullying environment, and very cliquey as well–

Katy: Oof, yeah!

Rory: ...which is odd to me, because you're there to work! You're there to help people! I think this kind of thing is more difficult when you're autistic but it's like, 'This is not a school! You're an adult!' And yeah, you can have work friendships, but why are you getting together to pull down another person? I just don't understand that. I see that happening so often. I'm the first one to be like, 'That's not acceptable' when it comes to somebody else but, when it's me, my body just freezes up. Having dissociative identity disorder as well, while I'm at work, I cannot switch. So you've just got so much going on, physically, psychologically, and then you're trying to be professional as well, and it's like, 'Oh my god, can we all just take a minute?'

Katy: Workplace bullies make things so much more stressful than it needs to be, for staff and for service users. I'm glad that you had that support from your bosses while you were working, at least.

What has been your own experience of living through the mental health system?

Rory: Well, that's a complex one, isn't it?! [Both laugh]

It's been pretty shocking. That's an understatement. It's shit. Especially in the past ten years, it's been terrible – the worst I've ever experienced, ever in my life. Living in these mental health rehabs, these hospitals, I can't even begin to describe it. It's gotten worse, even in the community. It's definitely traumatized me. I've been in bad places before this – my last placement was pretty bad – but I still got a lot from it. The place before that was horrific, and I've watched a lot of people lose their lives.

Before that, when I've been in my eating disorder treatment, community care, and the retreat in the unit for dissociative identity disorder, they were okay. The eating disorder treatment is a complex one, because I hate them, but they're good at their job! I'm not sure how much they helped me with my recovery, but at least they don't – psychologically, physically, or anything else – hurt you. The only bad thing is: they're making you do something you don't want to do, which is the whole point!

That doesn't mean that I've not had support from the mental health workers around me, because I have. I've had a wonderful psychologist and probably four great support workers, which I know is not a lot but it makes the world of difference. There are small positives to living here, like that I've got two hamsters now, but that wasn't down to my mental health team – I had to rescue them from other residents, so the hospital had to let me have them. I also feed the stray cats around here, when I can. The only other good thing in my mental health care is my social worker, and she's new – I've had two new ones in the past year.

My last resort of dealing with it being so bad in hospital is being so tired and 'not with it' enough that I don't really feel anything anymore. I feel like I have no personality left, which is funny to me, because I say that and I can just hear everyone being like, [disbelievingly] 'Excuse me...?!' [Both laugh] I just feel like I personally have no sense of self left, because I've had to use so much energy trying to survive here.

I don't have that many positive things. It's been very difficult and not very helpful. They don't really know what they're doing with me, or with anyone with complex needs, to be honest. It has the opportunity to be good – the whole mental health service has the opportunity to work well. It's just not using what it could use properly.

Katy: Why do you think that is?

Rory: I want to say money.

Katy: I was thinking that, too.

Rory: Yeah. I think it's funding. I think they messed up the funding so bad, a good few years back, that then they opted for cheaper 'alternative' treatments and underpaid health care workers, which means certain people are not invested in their job at all, which has made people more poorly, and then they're stuck in the system longer, and it all just goes round and round. And the 'quick treatment' counsellors and the support workers who don't actually work: they have an easy job, so they don't want to leave, so there's no vacancies for the good ones who actually want to help, and it just doesn't roll around into positives.

Katy: The bad health care workers always seem to stay, and the health care workers who want to make a difference always seem to cycle out. I've seen that a lot, too.

Rory: Yep! Yeah...

[There's a moment of silence, as if we're mourning.]

The government has a lot to answer for. I think a lot of private hospital directors and managers have a lot to answer for, too. Everyone's quick to say when one ward or unit is bad, but the system never changes, whether it's NHS or private. Each unit has a director that's in charge of what happens in that unit, but I think they all follow suit from others, and the same thing happens. If they make their own actual clinical decision as a director it might annoy a few people to rock the boat, but do you want the best for your patients and service users or not? I think there's a lot of different factors in play and now everyone's in a panic, so no one's doing anything until they're doing everything. The 'everything' is not important, because you don't need to paint the walls or buy new things – you need to focus on everything else.

Katy: Where would you put that money?

Rory: Where would I put, like, the 'wall painting money'?

Katy: Yeah, if you were the director of somewhere, where would you put the money?

Rory: First and foremost, I would completely revamp everything about health care workers. There needs to be so much change happening, but with health care workers first, because they're working immediately with service users. If you've got the right people working on the floor with service users, incidents will go down. Distress will go down. Feelings of loneliness and isolation will go down. If they're willing to go out on a walk with service users, go sit in the courtyard with them, and play a game with them, anything at all, that makes so much difference in a day. When you're on a unit – any sort of unit, even if you're in a general hospital – if you've got health care workers around you that engage with you, you can tell when there's a solid team of people. You can wake up and you're like, [energetic] 'Oh, it's this team!', and it's a happy feeling. But then some days, you wake up, and it's like, [defeated] 'Oh, it's this team...' And instantly, there is your day. They need to start from the bottom and go up – which maybe sounds backwards but, as somebody that's in these services, people need to be waking up and thinking, 'We're safe, we're supported, so I feel okay.' We don't need to be waking up and feeling like, 'I don't know who this is, they don't really talk to me,' or 'They're always rude to me,' or 'This team doesn't feel safe because they don't speak to any of us, they just sit in the corner and speak to each other.' There's a massive difference there. Even though people keep thinking we need to change the directors and the doctors, it needs to start with whoever sees the service users, because that's everything in mental health services. After that, build up from there.

Katy: It has me thinking back to when I was a mental health care worker in my early 20s. The number of times we would build a solid team on a unit, that got on well with each other and the service users; that was able to balance things really well and make sure everybody was getting what they needed; that made sure it was as safe, fun, and calm an atmosphere as possible...and then that team would get disbanded, because we were 'spending too much time with the residents instead of doing paperwork', or there was 'too much rapport'. It was awful for everyone.

Rory: A service user's home needs to feel like a home. Everybody knows the staff are not family but, right now, you're my family. I want to feel like we can sit down and we can have dinner, and then we can go and watch something. Some of us could play a game. Some of us could do some therapy work, some of us could go outside. If you've got a team that works well together, that's so much more confidently healing than a team that doesn't work together at all.

I never was the teacher's pet at school. I was the worst! But, in hospital, I'm the teacher's pet. I'm always the senior's favourite, so they're always my key worker. It used to really hurt me, because in one placement I would have all of my one-to-ones with the senior, who was my key worker, and she was running a team that didn't work with her or work with each other. I'd always watch her do everything ever. When you're a senior you have to come in early, you have to do security, you have to manage the team, you have to do timesheets, you have to do all of it while doing odd jobs, doing the levels, covering shifts, serving every meal, one-to-ones... It's not doable. It used to really upset me, and I wouldn't want to have my one-to-one because I'd be watching her run around like a lunatic, but then she'd come to me at the end of the day and be like, 'Please.' Then I'd think, 'You know what, she needs that time. Okay, yeah, let's go. We're not having it on the unit, though.' I'd take her off the unit and we'd go somewhere peaceful, and I wouldn't even need a one-to-one, we'd just do something. I'd watch her for like 11 hours, running around after everyone, and still coming to ask me if I needed anything at the end of the day. I'd want to take her away from there for a bit, even though she was always like, 'No, no, no, I'm taking you,' and I'd be like, 'Okay, I get it. You're taking me.'

It's always difficult to watch the genuinely good support workers get put into a bad team, because they then feel bad for not doing what they need to do. It's just such a difficult situation that really needs resolving, and – like I said – it needs to start with health care workers. They really are the backbone of any unit, I don't care what anyone says. They're around the service users 24/7 and, if they're not supported, then how can they support anyone else? They don't even just support service users – they support nurses, they support management with their notes, they do it all. I really think that needs to be focused on first.

Katy: I already agreed with you, but it's really sad to hear the effect that this has on you. There's so much that isn't being dealt with, here.

How would you like to see trauma being dealt with in a forensic mental health system?

Rory: Trauma-informed training needs to be given to everybody that works in a forensics setting. I mean everybody – everyone across the MDT (multidisciplinary team), even housekeeping. There's so many people that start the job and then, six months later, they're like, 'I've got my first training!' It's like, 'What do you mean! You've been here half a year!' But it's not their fault. It's not being offered to them, and they're being thrown into an environment where – for the most part, in forensic settings – trauma is one of the main causes that anybody is there.

Everyone needs to have a care plan that's fully focused on trauma alone. Usually in your care plans, you've got all these different sections labelled with numbers and letters, and then there's a subsection for trauma. There needs to be a completely separate care plan that's individualized. I know that nurses all up and down the country, if they could hear me, would be like, 'More care plans?!' [Both laugh] But I think the care plan needs to be formulated with a therapist that they've worked with in the community, if possible, alongside a psychologist that they work with inside the service, and then the nurse can input if they need to. I think it needs to be mental health professionals like therapists, psychologists, potentially occupational therapists, that formulate that plan. It doesn't even need to be a long plan, because this information should also be mentioned throughout their overall care plans, and again in their emergency planning. A separate plan would make the help they need more accessible.

I do think there needs to be more therapy offered, because there is just not enough. Again, I'm really lucky. I don't like saying that because I'm miserable here, but I have a very good forensic psychologist. I'm also seeing a very good private therapist, that I know I shouldn't have to have, because I shouldn't have to pay for this while I'm in hospital. If I didn't pay for my own therapist right now,

I would be on my own. I don't have anyone to speak to, here; nobody checks in on me. I have flashbacks, seizures, nightmares, all on my own, and nobody knows. I just think that, if there was something like a therapeutic check-in point every day, where someone could ask about any symptoms or anything that's happened, that would be so helpful. Even if service users don't want to do anything about how they're feeling, it would be helpful just to keep a log of it and monitor it – because they don't monitor these things. The staff just deal with behaviours when it affects them, and then hope the cause goes away. Nothing comes from it. They just ignore it, and then you're just left to deal with it. They're not very in touch with service users and what they need.

I also think it would be helpful if there were more therapeutic groups running out there, both outpatient and inpatient, that had properly trauma-informed facilitators. That would make a lot of difference because, right now, it just seems like most forensic inpatient and outpatient services are recognizing that these people have trauma, but then just smoothing things over until they can't ignore it anymore. It is not very progressive.

Katy: It is not how trauma works – it doesn't smooth over.

Rory: No. It's not okay. Things like therapy groups should be offered consistently so that people are given that opportunity to work through their trauma. These groups used to be around 15 years ago but I do not hear about any of that any more. That's probably due to budget cuts, and they haven't even put anything as a replacement for that. I worry about those that relied on those groups, because what are they doing now? Probably in hospitals and not well, and not getting that treatment.

I don't really know what can be done, but I do know that not enough is being done at all. It's really rough in mental health services in general. I've been lucky with some of the trauma care I've received, but I think I've been traumatized more in hospitals than helped by them. It's a bit of an odd balance for me.

Katy: It's awful, as well, because what you're talking about here should be the bare minimum of care – that somebody checks in on you and asks how you're doing, that everyone has appropriate training, that help is offered. That's what being in hospital is supposed to be. When you're in the forensic system, that's the care you deserve.

Rory: It's just not doable here, though, it is? I'm kind of used to it. I look after myself. I just eat my ice pops and stop to feed the stray cats. That has to be enough for now.

Katy: I'm glad that you have these small things, and also it's definitely not enough.

What would you say to LGBTQ+ people who want to study and work in mental health?

Rory: The OU feels like a great choice for both the LGBTQ+ community, and the neurodivergent community, and both entwined. There's so many different groups, and they run sessions like coffee mornings on the tutorial site. They have evening game nights and quizzes. It's so good! That's not even to do with your studies, but it's that connection that's important. Especially given that the course is online, you can feel a little bit disconnected from the people you've studied with, so these things help you get to know other people. I've met some wonderful people, and you're supported by all the tutors, and I've had nothing but positive experiences. The OU is so good when it comes to anything neurodiverse and LGBTQ+, anything at all. You can get the support that you need in any area.

Now, in terms of working in the mental health field – again, I don't necessarily have a negative or positive view. Everyone's always been quite supportive of my sexuality. I'm just wary of it, because

I think about how much I used to mask and not speak to anybody about anything to do with my identity or my personal life. Nobody's ever made comments about my sexuality or anything like that, but I think that's probably because – for the most part – people just didn't know. Which was odd, because I'm so gay! [Both laugh]

The one thing that I would always say is, make sure that you've got somebody above you that you can go to if somebody else makes your identity a problem. It probably won't happen but, if you have somebody that you trust above you that you can go to, you will feel safer if anybody ever tries to bully you. It's always better for your health and your mind-set to have an advocate at work because, if something does happen, I wouldn't want anybody to ever feel alone with that.

I have found that, over the years, it's gotten a lot better. I really do think a good few years ago, when I started this work, it would not have been as inclusive at all. It's not perfect now, but it's a lot better than it was. For the most part, I find the work quite inclusive, and I know places like the NHS have LGBTQ+ groups these days in the workplace.

Unfortunately, not everyone around you will be a nice person. I have had to stand up to people when I've heard them make comments about others' sexuality – when it's not about me, and it's not to me, I make sure I say something. Colleagues can always surprise you – the same as every situation, really. Being safe from others, emotionally, physically, in every way, should always be everyone's priority, but it shouldn't have to be.

Katy: What would you say to LGBTQ+ people who are currently trying to heal within the mental health system?

Rory: You've got to keep going. You've already been through enough – no matter what that is, in any capacity. You've already been through enough, and you need to keep going.

Work alongside anything that's working alongside you. It can be anything you care about. You can't work alongside something that's working against you but, if you find yourself in that position, you can always work alongside yourself. You can trust yourself to look after yourself, because you've already lived through so much.

It's all doable. It's going to be rubbish, but it's doable.

I'm sorry if these were bad answers, by the way, but these were my honest answers.

Katy: There are no bad answers because you are inherently worth listening to. I think that mental health writing needs more honesty, more congruence, from the people working in it and living in it.

Rory: Non-fiction mental health books seem fictional sometimes. People want treatment and recovery to be so great, so they write about it in a romanticized way because this is what we want, and they think you don't need to know what it actually is, only what it should be.

Katy: I guess people want to show that there's hope?

Rory: Mental health doesn't have to be hopeful – sometimes, it's just shit. But, sometimes, I feel like there's a lot of hope to hold on to. Even while things are really crap, I'm hopeful. I'm hopeful for others. Anybody can survive. People can do it. Especially if you can find a good place, and good people, to support you, you can do it.

Katy's post-interview thoughts

While I wanted this book to offer hope to everyone who reads it, in Rory's words, 'Mental health doesn't have to be hopeful.' This interview might be tough reading, as Rory talks frankly about both the help and the despair they have found in the hands of the psychiatric system, but I often tell my clients that we have to recognize the hard parts so that things can get better. The pain found here is not an isolated incident, and attention must be paid by all of us so that we can work together to change things. I've found hope in Rory herself, in the strength she shows every day, and in her fight for a better future for those in forensic and psychiatric systems. I hope that you can find that hope here, too.

If you'd like to know more

Bent Bars. A UK-based letter-writing project connecting LGBTQ+ prisoners and detainees to penpals outside prison. The project includes people who are held in prisons, secure mental health units, and immigration detention. www.bentbarsproject.org

Mad or Bad? A Critical Approach to Counselling and Forensic Psychology, edited by Andreas Vossler, Catriona Havard, Graham Pike, Meg-John Barker, and Bianca Raabe, 2017. Created by several experts at the Open University, this book offers a wide and deep examination of forensic therapeutic practices in the UK, including research into how sexuality, gender, and experiences of oppression are tied in with our beliefs around who is 'mad' and who is 'bad'.

Care Work: Dreaming Disability Justice, by Leah Lakshmi Piepzna-Samarasinha, 2018. This book features a collection of essays that centre disability justice, encouraging us to push for power, community, and inclusion for all sick and disabled people. I'd recommend it to everyone, though I think it's especially urgent reading for anyone working in the mental health and caring professions.

Queer Healing with Lucy Fox

An introduction to Lucy

Lucy (she/they) was a queer, transfeminine, non-binary trans woman in her 40s, who had lived with the consequences of forced conversion therapy since her early 20s. She was neurodivergent in many ways – she was autistic and ADHD, which brought complicated joy and difficulty to her life, and she also lived with brain damage after being subjected to ECT (electroconvulsive therapy) as part of conversion therapy, which only brought grief and pain. After battling with the mental health system in England for her whole life, she was on the path towards continued training as a therapist in order to provide other LGBTQ+ people with the kind of care she should have always received.

Conversion therapy – sometimes known as 'reparative therapy' – is the abusive pseudoscientific practice of trying to alter somebody's LGBTQ+ identity, including (but certainly not limited to) such historical and present methods as 'praying the gay away' (Strudwick, 2011), withheld gender-related health care (Wright, Candy, and King, 2018), aversion treatment (Spandler and Carr, 2022), lobotomies (Kaye, 2023), GET – also known as gender exploratory reparative therapy (Ashley, 2023), and much more (Blakemore, 2023).

Conversion therapy is unnecessary and ineffective, and it causes lasting damage no matter the method (Turban *et al.*, 2020).

At the time I am writing this introduction to Lucy's interview, conversion therapy is still legally practised in the UK (Toesland, Gross, and Nikolaeva, 2023). It's become an increasingly discussed topic while I've worked as a therapist, often to the distress of queer therapists and queer clients alike. The developments have not often been good – for example, during the time in which I conducted this interview, a UK-based registering body for psychotherapists, the UKCP (United Kingdom Council for Psychotherapy), divested from its long-term commitment to ending conversion therapy by taking 'the decision to withdraw its signature from the *Memorandum of Understanding on Conversion Therapy in the UK* v2 (MoU) and its membership of the Coalition Against Conversion Therapy' (UKCP, 2023). I also know several trans people who worry that the UK Supreme Court ruling in 2025 – that trans people are not legally protected as their true genders – may also leave trans people more vulnerable to conversation therapy. In a time where conversion therapy is an increasingly discussed topic, survivors' voices like Lucy's need to be prioritized.

Lucy and I were married the year before I interviewed her for this book. As of the beginning of 2025, we'd been together for nearly eight healing and adventure-filled years. In April 2025, Lucy passed away as a result of bigotry and violence, both in her personal life and at large in the UK.

Lucy's interview

Lucy: I'm Lucy. I am a transfem non-binary person. I'm 45, I'm married, and I live in the northeast of England.

I feel like I don't resonate with any particular gender. It all feels a bit strange, like the programming doesn't fit. Like society's gone,

'Here's a gender!' and I've gone, [like she's trying to be polite about a terrible present] 'Yeah, let's put that away somewhere and try to never think about it again...!' [Katy laughs] So, I don't particularly feel like any gender but, when I see my inner self, I see myself as having a body like somebody AFAB (assigned female at birth). Sometimes I describe myself as a non-binary trans woman. I'm more comfortable in femme-presenting roles, although I tend to not pay much attention to things like feminine stereotypes or what fashion women are supposed to wear. Being neurodivergent, I miss a lot of the social things that most people seem to understand.

Katy: I think you're very stylish.

Lucy: Thank you. I just wear what I feel comfortable in, most of the time. Mostly looking femme makes me feel the most comfortable, but I don't particularly fall under any persuasion when it comes to clothing these days. I don't feel like I have to present in any particular way, certainly not for the benefit of society.

Katy: Anything else you want to say about who you are or what you've done?

Lucy: I think my life has been pretty boring, to be honest, in terms of achievements. I haven't really achieved a great deal.

Katy: You've achieved so much!

Lucy: I suppose it depends how you define achievements. For me, just surviving has been probably my biggest achievement, up there with marrying my amazing wife.

Katy: Hey, that's me!

Lucy: It is you! [Katy laughs. A cat meows plaintively in the distance.] And the cats have reminded me that I'm a cat mum.

Katy: The cats have been trying to break into my office again today. They're desperate to be part of these interviews!

So, you were a queer, trans, neurodivergent person coming of age in the 1980s and 90s. What was that like for you?

Lucy: For me, it kind of came in two flavours.

There was not much positive LGBTQ+ representation around me, in particular for trans people. Gay people were described as people to avoid, because they were thought to be predators. Being queer had that societal feel of being terrifying, especially with people being murdered and beaten left, right, and centre for being gay.

But as an individual who didn't particularly present as gay, or at least wasn't 'clocked' until my teens, it was pretty inconsequential until it affected me directly. It affected me basically from high school onwards, which is why I didn't attend my last two years – it was a dangerous, scary place. Being seen as queer made me such a huge target and, being someone who was clocked as queer in those days, people would not come to your defence. It was a very lonely and scary time growing up in terms of sexuality and gender, which caused me to repress a lot of my sexuality, and my gender as well.

Katy: I remember being a kid in the 1990s and 'gay' being the ultimate slur on the playground.

Lucy: It was very much like that. That doesn't seem to have changed too much between our two generations (Gen X and millennial). Online, now, it still seems like 'woke' and 'trans' are some of the ultimate insults. What was I called the other day? 'A liberal lefty snowflake.' I guess gayness is still implied there as an insult, but maybe it's not as predominantly dangerous as it was in my time, or your time.

I think that's changing, especially as now you tend to find that gay children will have more chance of having a social group of their own who will stick up for them and use their voices, which is something you would never see in my day, at all, ever. I think that would probably not have been likely in your day, either?

Katy: When I was a kid, I didn't have many friends. I had a lot of figuring out to do as a kid about my gender and my sexuality, mostly because of societal stuff, like living under Section 28 (a law in effect from 1988 to 2003 in England, Scotland, and Wales that made 'promoting homosexuality' illegal in schools, meaning LGBTQ+ identities and lives could not be discussed and supportive LGBTQ+ literature was banned), and the general homophobia and trans hostility of the time. I did have a few friends, though, and as an adult, all of those friends have turned out to be queer in some way. So it's interesting, because I feel like I did have a queer social circle, but none of us knew, none of us were out. None of us had figured that out when we were all hanging out, but we still somehow came together. I am hoping that – and it seems like – young people today have more of a chance of having an out and supportive queer social circle.

Lucy: I absolutely agree. I think going back to my school years, there weren't queer circles. Groups were divided in different ways – the cool kids, the not-so-cool kids, the poor kids and the council estate kids, the swots, it was all that kind of thing. There was never a sexuality divide because people did not admit to it and, if anyone looked, acted, or said anything that could be construed as gay, it was a target on your back. Being perceived as gay was something all the kids could rally around, even the groups who hated each other. It was not fun being the rallying cry for the violence of an entire school. [Lucy laughs sadly]

Katy: No, it never feels good to be the pariah.

Lucy: Especially when even teachers pretend not to see things because you're the queer kid. I imagine it's easier to keep the school as a whole under control when you're not protecting the pariah. Teachers don't want to give up that control.

Katy: It's classic scapegoating.

Lucy: 'Let's not admit our mistakes – we'll point at the queer kid, instead.' Or I suppose, these days, it's the trans kid. [Lucy starts leaning away from the camera, out of view]

Katy: Sure. Speaking of, I – oh, where have you gone? Are you okay?

Lucy: [Lucy's head pops back into the frame. She's rubbing gel on one arm] I'm sorry, I forgot to put my hormone gel on this morning and this reminded me. I do apologize.

Katy: No, it's okay!

Lucy: The privileges of being a transfem.

Katy: I'm absolutely going to put this in the book. This is gold.

Lucy: [Lucy laughs] That's fine! What were you going to say?

Katy: Part of your experience as a young, queer, transfem person was going through conversion therapy. Do you want to tell me about that?

Lucy: I preface this by saying: a lot of the memories I have are jarred and blurry from that time, and my memory since has not been amazing. I have quite significant memory problems and brain damage from conversion therapy.

I will have been about 19 years old, so this was in the 1990s. I was taken to a psychiatric unit in Scunthorpe (UK), because I had taken an overdose and I tried to fight off the policeman who was trying to save my life. I was cuffed, taken to hospital, and released into Ward 18, which was a psychiatric unit. The psychiatric unit was full, so I was transferred to another psychiatric unit that was affiliated with, but not run by, the NHS. This was a very Catholic-run unit and, unfortunately for me, one of their specialities was conversion therapy to 'cure' people of being gay or trans. [Lucy pauses to take some deep breaths]

Katy: It's okay. Please take your time. Remember, only talk about what you want to talk about.

Lucy: I know. I think it's important to get things like this out, though, to show people the actual reality of it.

It's very disjointed, from here. There were a few other people on the ward with me who were going through the same treatment. When we'd come back from the ECT, we would sit around each other and tell each other things about the person who was coming back, to help them reconnect to their memories, because we were all finding our memories were getting quite disturbed. We couldn't remember certain things. We had almost a mini-support group within the ward who were trying to combat the effects of ECT for each other.

The things that are most prominent in my memory are the sounds. There was always music – either Catholic music, or hymns, or Bible readings, or readings of prayers. We'd have to pray a lot.

We were very restricted on what we were allowed to eat. I think I lost 2 stone when I was on the ward, and I was only there for about three months, I think. That's how long I think I was there, anyway – I have no memory of the passing of time there, and no way to confirm. There weren't clocks or anything, and we weren't allowed mobile phones or watches, so there was no way to know the time. So, we never really knew the time of day, and that was horrendous in itself.

The other most prominent memories are being on the chair where they did the ECT. There was nothing else in the room except for the chair and the ECT equipment, and the whole place was a very white, sterile environment. It was almost like a dentist's chair, and they leant you back in it, and they strapped your arms and legs and your chest to the table. Then they put things like boxing mouth-guards in your mouth, and then they attached wires to you. Then, you'd convulse violently against the restraints for however long – I've no idea what the time frame was. It could have been minutes, it could have been hours; I had no way to tell.

The ECT was horrific. It was torture. I felt like parts of me were being torn away – parts of my identity and who I am. I was fighting to grasp parts of who I am, but it was like trying to catch fog; I just couldn't. No matter what I did, there was nothing I could do to try and keep a lot of the memories they tried to make me lose, so a lot of my memories are really disjointed. It terrifies me, because there are things I know I've forgotten that are important things in my life and, when you really cut everything else away, we are a sum of our experiences, our memories. When you take those memories away, you take away from the whole, from the person. You lose yourself.

Katy: It sounds like that was the point.

Lucy: Yes. It was horrific. I wouldn't wish that on my worst enemy. I wouldn't wish that on anyone, ever. It is inhumane. You wouldn't do that to an animal, because you would go to jail, but it's okay to do it to someone who's gay or trans. It's still not illegal in the UK, so it's not just torture – it's government-sanctioned torture.

Katy: Did you know that, recently, at least one of the 'major league' psychotherapeutic governing bodies have pulled out of their commitment to banning conversion therapy for everyone? It absolutely disgusts me. It really scares me.

Lucy: It's horrifying because, every time you go into therapy as an LGBTQ+ person, you go in with a fear that they may want you to go through conversion therapy. That fear will last until it's illegal.

How can anyone propose to be someone who is offering a therapeutic healing experience while torturing people? And conversion therapy is internationally regarded as torture! But our government's like, 'Hmm, maybe it's not!'

Katy: Trans people are often pathologized in psychiatric care and, clearly, this has been the case for you in terms of conversion therapy. How do you think that being trans and queer has affected the support that you've been able to access?

Lucy: That has been a major barrier to me receiving mental health care.

I currently have a diagnosis of EUPD, or emotionally unstable personality disorder (which is known as BPD, or borderline personality disorder, outside the UK). This coincided with the time I was being assessed for autism by a team who said that I have zero autistic traits – even though I had already been diagnosed with autism – and that their recommendation would be a personality disorder diagnosis. I personally believe all of this is because of my gender. I believe, absolutely, that all of this is 100% down to my gender and nothing else, because I have seen psychiatrists since then who have said that my emotional regulation, the way I deal with conflict, and the way I work with my emotions does not meet the criteria of EUPD. For example, I don't jump from the lowest to the highest emotional points like they said I did in the meetings;

I was just angry that I was being messed around by mental health services, and I don't present in a 'typically AMAB (assigned male at birth) autistic' way, so they decided I was a hysterical woman instead.

Now, because I have an EUPD diagnosis, which is a tier-four mental health diagnosis – the most severe diagnosis that can be offered by the NHS – I am no longer allowed to access about 90% of non-private mental health support, because people are not trained to work with really poorly people. These mental health workers often do not want to take the training, and their managers do not want to take the expense of the training and the insurance, which means I am *persona non grata* from so much support. And, again, this is rooted in my gender.

Katy: As a therapist, this is something that I've heard from trans people, and especially from trans people who are seen as women, over and over again. Research shows that there is so much overlap and misdiagnosis of traumatized autistic people, and traumatized neurodivergent people in general, who are misdiagnosed as having EUPD.

One of the things that really gets me about this – that I've heard from clients, and that I've seen directly as you've tried to look for help in the past – is that one of the things that backs up someone having an EUPD diagnosis is when you try to counteract that diagnosis. If you get angry about the diagnosis, or upset about the way the mental health system has treated you, they'll say it's because you have EUPD.

Lucy: Yes, that is something I have run into multiple times. I remember one specific incident – and this is before we met, I believe, although I'm not 100% certain because my memory, again, is absolutely horrific. (We had actually met at this point, because I remember this happening, but we were still in an early, long-distance era of our relationship, so I wasn't there in person.) I was under the care of a local community mental health team. I was seeing one of the doctors, and I was explaining why I wanted to challenge the diagnosis. As I was explaining it, he was basically telling me I had to shut up and listen to why that diagnosis meets my 'symptoms'. So I gave him space, and I listened to him say his piece, and then I tried to say again, 'No, that isn't accurate, and this is why I don't feel I have it.' Then my support worker at the time, who was supposed to support me, said, 'You need to listen to the doctor. Your opinion about it doesn't matter, because the doctor is the professional.' This is embarrassing for me to admit, but I had a bad meltdown in the office after that, and I had to get back to my safe place, which was my home with my cat. I was in so much of a panic that I ran through traffic – I nearly got run over – and I eventually made it home, locked the door, and I just couldn't see anyone or talk to anyone because I was in such a heavy state of meltdown. I had that meltdown because I didn't have a voice: no one was advocating for me, no one would listen to me. Because I'm autistic, and because I'm anxious, and because of the ECT and the trauma around that, I really struggled to advocate for myself.

It wasn't until you – my wife – came onto the scene and started advocating for me that I was taken seriously. Because I suddenly had someone with me who could say, 'Actually, no, she's right. This is what she says and here is the evidence you need,' people listened. There were fewer people telling me to shut up and listen to the doctor, and treating me like I'm just a silly crazy person.

Katy: Those experiences were horrible. I knew that people were only listening because I was accompanying you to your appointments carefully dressed like a perfect, professional, cis-appearing person, and making sure everyone knew I had psychiatric knowledge and experience, and that I was going to be paying close attention to how professionals treated you. I just said everything that you had been saying, and I watched everyone suddenly pay attention. It made me so angry.

Lucy: It wasn't a great point. Don't get me wrong – I was absolutely grateful to you on so many levels, because you have been the strongest support I've had in my life, and it's constant support.

Katy: Thank you.

Lucy: But it was also so traumatic to watch something I've been saying for years and years and years suddenly be taken seriously. All because they thought a cis person was saying it.

That crushes something inside you. You lose faith in humanity and in compassion. These are supposed to be people who are professionals to support you, and help you, and provide mental health support. I left them more broken than when I went in.

Katy: It's a common story, unfortunately.

Lucy: I've had to pay, and you've paid for me, to have six years of private therapy, and I will say at least a year or two of that was undoing the damage that the NHS has done. It's not been one or two incidents; it is a repeated pattern of behaviour over a consistent number of, not just years, but decades.

Trying to access mental health support when I was 20 was absolutely ridiculous. When I was released from the Catholic ward, they had community workers who were supposed to be a mental health transit to get you to the right service. The trouble was, I spent three years under community workers who would see me once a month and say 'How are you feeling? Fill out this form. We're still looking for the right therapy pathway for you. See you next month.'

Katy: I know clients who have had similar treatment now.

Lucy: The system needs to change. I mean, there's still such a horrendous fear around the NHS mental health system because of their predisposition to sectioning people instead of supporting and helping people in their community. The worry is that they'll either ignore you or lock you away. What they seem to still be saying to the world is, 'We don't care about the person who's struggling with their mental health. We'll label them crazy. We'll put them in a place somewhere we can ignore them and society doesn't have to see it.'

It's almost like it's too much of an embarrassment to society to see someone has some mental health problems. I think that's changing for younger people, but it's changing slowly. I know trans people often really worry about how the mental health system will treat them, but it's not just bad for trans people – there is still this systemic embarrassment and fear of mental health problems for everyone. An example is how cis and trans men still have this horrendous toxic attitude forced upon them that they are not allowed to cry, or have emotions beyond anger and rage.

Katy: I see how that affects trans men and transmasculine people in my therapy office all the time.

Lucy: I know transmasculine friends who have been told they're too emotional to transition. I've had transmasc friends, and agender friends who are AFAB (assigned female at birth) and present in a masculine way, tell me how much struggle they've had with necessary things like mastectomies. Even people in their 30s and 40s, they're having to fight and argue and jump through hoops to get a mastectomy, or to have other operations and treatments that are beneficial, because they've struggled with things like depression in the past. Doctors don't even take into account that dysphoria can be depressing. So many of us trans people are traumatized from the current experience of being trans in this society – of course we tend to have more mental illness!

Transmascs also have to deal with that whole thing of, like, 'Oh, you're not actually a trans man. You're just a lesbian dressed as a dude. You've been abused and groomed into wanting to change. You must be delusional.'

Katy: I've seen that, especially if there's any neurodivergence in their medical history, it's always used against people when it comes to transitioning.

Lucy: Oh, god, yeah. [Sarcastically] Because autistic people can't know what they want!

It makes me so angry when people are like, 'You're trans and you have trauma? Then you mustn't be valid. If you're traumatized you're not really trans, you're just escaping yourself.' Escaping what, into what? I mean, I'm not being a dick about it, but being trans has been one of the hardest things I've had to go through in my life, if not the hardest thing. And that includes the time I was clinically dead for three seconds.

Katy: What has it been like for you now, seeking and finding good mental health support as a traumatized queer person? What has that looked like for you?

Lucy: For me, I always seem to think of this as there being two sides – Pre-Wife, and Post-Wife.

Pre-Wife, in my early 30s, I had a lot of connections within the trans community. I was an activist. I worked as a suicide and crisis prevention worker, specifically for trans youths. I've done a lot of work like that, and I have connections, but even having those connections, finding therapists locally who were neurodivergent-aware, trans-aware, sexuality-aware, and the various things that come with that, was a nightmare.

It's so hard to find mental health people that meet the specific criteria you need when you're queer and neurodivergent. If you think of it like a pyramid, you've got all the therapists at the bottom. The next layer up, you've got the ones who are neuro-affirming. The next layer, they're good with neurodivergent clients and they're trained in non-straight sexuality. The next layer has the ones who offer all that, plus gender. Now you've got this tiny, tiny little bit at the top to pick from, which is only a handful of therapists, and then just having a few therapists who are trained in all that doesn't mean you'll have the therapeutic relationship you want with all of them – you need to have a beneficial and healthy therapeutic experience, which isn't guaranteed. You could try everyone in that handful and not have a connection with any of them. So, then, you're like, 'Okay, so I'll have to step down a level. I'll try someone who's not any good with trans stuff, but is good with the other things.' You end up having to pick and choose which bits of you need the most attention, and which therapist is going to provide the most support where you don't have to be your therapist's educator. For me, that feels like it changes the dynamic of the therapeutic relationship substantially.

Katy: Yeah, god, having to do 'Gender 101' with your therapist is so soul sucking.

Lucy: I've had that experience too many times – Gender 101, Sexuality 101, Ethical Non-Monogamy 101, BDSM 101, Neurodivergence 101... Having to explain neurodivergence to therapists is particularly draining because there *isn't* a Neurodivergence 101. It encompasses so many things and, even in one area like brain damage or autism or ADHD, it's so expansive. There's so many different presentations of neurodivergence. I mean, me and you have such different neurodivergent traits, and we're both very neurodivergent, often with the same labels, just often in completely different ways.

Katy: So then, what was your experience like after we met? In the last six-ish years, what has it been like trying to find good mental health support?

Lucy: It's actually been massively beneficial having my wife around, because I struggle with trying to find resources, now, and trying to make connections, and trying to work out what's best for me. It's embarrassing to admit that. I get really indecisive because I struggle with my thought processes a lot. My wife coming in to my life has been amazing because they're very organized and good at providing these resources. I'll talk about how I need to see a therapist, and you'll ask if I need help, and then you'll go, 'Here's a list of therapists that might be of benefit or interest in my opinion,' and then I can winnow the list down. You're very good at that.

Katy: I try.

Lucy: You do provide amazing resources, and these are resources that I wouldn't have been able to access without you, as a trans person, despite these resources often being aimed at trans people. These things are not as easy to find in the ways that I am used to.

I don't think it's the done thing to advertise your trans support in mental health circles, especially in this day and age, and increasingly with things like the Cass Review, Tavistock shutting down, how some people responded to the murder of Brianna Ghey, all these horrible things that we have to watch others cheer for. They create an environment where any sort of trans positivity is immediately shut down, and the major media providers only show negative lies about trans people. So, I think trans-positive health spaces are often under the radar to avoid being shut down or bullied by people who are anti-trans.

You've been able to find some great therapy options for me, though.

Katy: What do you think makes somebody a good therapist for someone like you?

Lucy: There are boxes to tick that have different levels of importance. Obviously at the top for me, someone who is trans-aware. I spend all of my life explaining my gender to everyone, all the time. I don't want to go into therapy and do it again. It becomes rote, you know? You end up reading the script, you've done it so many times. It's boring and it's disheartening. So, obviously, someone who is trans-aware, and also someone who is neurodivergence-aware, because I don't want to explain my neurodivergence over and over again. Someone who is aware of different relationship dynamics and styles is also important to me.

A good therapist needs to be someone who is compassionate and wants to have a therapeutic relationship of equals, where I don't feel like I'm being spoken down to by the professional. Being condescended to feels prohibitive in a healing relationship. It's hard for me to open up to someone who takes that authoritative 'I am the professional and you are just the client' role. I understand that they *are* the professional, but I need someone who will make me feel more on their level as an equal, so I can share with an equal.

Katy: I agree that there has to be power in both of those roles. A therapist might be an expert in therapy, but you are always going to be the expert in you, and what you need, and who you are.

Lucy: One of my biggest bugbears is when I don't feel acknowledged in a therapeutic relationship. I hate that feeling when a therapist basically says, 'I can see why you feel that way, but it's wrong. You shouldn't feel that way.' I much prefer someone who says something like, 'I can see you are feeling this, and that's affecting you in a certain way. What does that mean to you? Am I correct there? Is there more you want to add?' If they ask further questions in a way that doesn't make it feel like I'm doing something wrong, then I will open up. Do the opposite, and I will close down.

I believe you had an experience like that with a past therapist, when you were told you weren't allowed to express a feeling, and you shut down to the therapist?

Katy: Yeah, I was in my 20s and the therapist said they didn't like it when I expressed my low self-esteem, and that made me completely shut down. It didn't feel like a safe place to talk about how I was feeling any more.

Lucy: That energy is so damaging, which is why acknowledging what the person is saying and being empathetic to it is so important.

Katy: Totally. Would you like to tell me about your experiences of being a neurodivergent, trans, queer person who's looking for counselling training?

Lucy: It's both exciting and daunting. It's exciting because I enjoy learning things about psychology and the workings of the brain. I also have this desire to help people heal, to help the world, and to help people feel better. I've worked as a crisis counsellor before and I was good at my job, and I loved it. Practising therapy is something that I think would benefit both me and other people. It's something I'm definitely excited to do.

But being a transfem who is neurodivergent and not able-bodied adds a bunch of different elements that makes it quite scary. I'm going to be training on a campus with people who are therapists, which I'm assuming will be fine, but the people who aren't therapists on the campus may react in a less empathetic way. There's also the fear that people within the therapeutic experience, who are training with me, may also react in a negative way because I am disabled, because I am neurodivergent, because I am trans, because I am most obviously, definitely queer. That's a lot of potential trigger points for people to attack me and, not being able-bodied, it's not like I can physically defend myself against an attack. That adds that element of fear. There's also the brain damage from the ECT. Sometimes, I forget things. What if I forget things during a therapy session? What if I forget things while I'm doing an exam and I fail? What if my brain just won't take the information in because of the damage done by the ECT? There's all these little things going around that I'll have to try and balance.

There's also being in therapy while learning therapy skills, which then adds the complication of basically everything we've talked about already with finding a therapist. That adds another layer of need to the pyramid; it makes it an even tighter, smaller triangle at the top, because then you have to find ones who understand you *and* who will see therapy students *and* who are accredited with the association that the education body that provides the training wants you to be with, and if you can't, that can then exclude you from the training and from education. So, therapy is once again a barrier – or rather, my being trans is a barrier to having therapy, which is a barrier to my potential career.

Katy: I know that when I was training to be a therapist – when I'd been out as some flavour of queer for a long time but I was just a wee babytrans – I had to have a UKCP-registered therapist that was local, so I could see them face-to-face, and also working within my modality. That really limited the kinds of therapist I could see. I ended up with therapists who weren't knowledgeable about who I was and what I was bringing to sessions. My therapist when I lived in the Midlands (UK) was very good despite all of that, but it also meant that another therapist I saw during my training did not understand who I was at all.

Lucy: Unfortunately, I can absolutely relate to that. I have had therapists who have just not got it, who have misgendered me repeatedly despite being reminded.

My psychiatrist for my early gender transition misgendered me repeatedly, and told me that my ambition to work as a therapist was beyond my means, and I should have a more realistic goal like maybe being a manager of a grocery store. He said he didn't think I should transition because I was disabled and, at the time, unemployed, and that the only reason I was being put forward for transition-related services was because he was leaving and didn't have to care anymore.

Katy: You've definitely proved that guy wrong. What has your work in the mental health field been like so far?

Lucy: I have had an interesting array of experience in mental health, both as a practitioner and client. I've worked with several charities that help suicidal people, including the Samaritans. It's been mainly online, rather than in person.

The role I'm maybe most proud of was as a crisis worker, through a community called *Laura's Playground* (a once well-regarded but sadly now defunct online forum for trans people), which used to be the only place you could find online that provided trained, accredited crisis support and suicide prevention for people like myself. We all had to go through the same training and learn all the same things, and we all had to have our accreditation before we were allowed to work. It was strictly monitored and regulated. We provided support to so, so, so many trans people. Predominantly, I would say 60–70% of the people coming in were young transmasculine people. At the time there was a common theme of young transmasc people who were not respected by their parents, and told they were some form of tomboy, and forced to 'act like girls'.

We tried to provide as much support to them, to everyone, as possible, but we were limited. We were a limited resource providing limited support in a limited capacity. With mental health services that are low in funds, you can't help everyone. We hit limit after limit, and then you get to the bottom with the tiny percentage that you can help. I know what it's like to be someone who's desperate for help, and I really, really tried to help. It's awful when you get your hands tied at every turn.

Katy: You help so many people, then and now. I'm proud of you.

Lucy: I'm proud of the ones I've helped. I feel nothing but the deepest sympathy for all those trans youths, and trans adults, and queer people out there, who aren't getting the support, who don't have the networks, and who don't have access to the therapists they need. There are so many barriers to good mental health, whether it be monetary, social, accessibility-based, and more. The worst part for me is being on the inside, seeing those barriers, and feeling powerless to do anything about them.

Katy: I totally get that. It's horrible seeing how vulnerable queer people are right now, especially trans people, and knowing that it's that vulnerability that often keeps people from therapy. That vulnerability and oppression means we're less likely to be helped in NHS services, and also we're less likely to have the money to seek private therapy.

Lucy: Right. From the inside, when you're something like a crisis worker or a care worker, and you're watching that, you feel almost complicit because you're part of the system that is discriminating against these minorities, and you can't change it. You've got to live by that system and, if you step out of that system, then the system takes away your power to help.

Katy: I really feel you there. I have yet to find a way to not be crushed by that system.

Lucy: I see you try really hard to not be complicit.

Katy: I was thinking especially about our ongoing discussion about the rates that I charge as a therapist. I know you think I don't charge a high enough rate, and you're probably right, but then I end up in this horrible cycle of oppression when I think about raising my fees. I don't charge as much as I maybe should, because most of my clients are trans or other flavours of queer and they don't make a lot of money, but then, in not charging as much as I should, I'm also a trans queer person who's not making a lot of money. I don't know how to step out of that system.

Lucy: [Rhetorical] And where does it end? Where does that spiral end?

Katy: What coping techniques have you learned to help with your mental health?

Lucy: Do you want the good, the bad, or the ugly?

Katy: Let's do the 'bad' first, and then the 'good'.

Lucy: Okay. Some of my worst coping techniques have revolved around self-harm. That's been cutting, having too-hot baths, depriving myself, various other methods. I've now been self-harm free for seven years.

Cannabis had been used significantly to numb myself from the pain of life. All of this is because, when you can't get support like therapy, you rely on what's left. I smoked weed instead. It helped me to dissociate.

Disassociation has been a heavily used coping technique for me as well, in the negative bracket, and it's caused a lot of emotional damage, because it's taken me a long time to reconnect to my emotions and to feel them as fully as I do. That was probably the mainstay of my more negative 'Pre-Wife' coping techniques.

Katy: What do you think has been helpful?

Lucy: There are very different layers of support that have been beneficial and, I would say, pivotal to my current coping techniques. The most important has been having healthy relationships with the people around me – my wife, my friends and family, even neighbours. Being able to open myself up and be vulnerable with them, and have myself be supported and not shown disdain or negativity.

The constant support from my wife has been phenomenal. I've never experienced support like it, and they have been the mainstay of my recovery and my mental health battles in the last six years. They also helped me find amazing therapists. I've had so much amazing therapy, which has been life altering for me.

With all this new support, my emotions are more organic; they're more natural; they flow freely from me; and I feel them fully. It's not always great – I lost my dad in October. I'm still grieving through that, but before, I would have smoked, or done something horrendous to myself, and shut down. Now, I cry. I talk about my dad. I get support. I sometimes listen to some of his favourite songs, and I feel what I feel, and I process that feeling in the moment – or, as 'in the moment' as it gets with me being a neurodivergent person who has a fair bit of lag between incident and feeling, sometimes. I feel like processing time can often be longer for neurodivergent people, but it can also feel longer in me than for other neurodivergent people, too. That's not that I'm saying I'm more neurodivergent than anyone else, it's just that specific thing takes me longer than most people.

Katy: Maybe, but that's a difficult skill to learn when it doesn't come naturally, or when it's been traumatized out of you.

Lucy: It's definitely been traumatized out of me through the years. If I told you the life story of my trauma, you may never recover! [Lucy laughs] But I'm still here. And, despite the years, the homelessness, the fight for my mental health, I am happy. I'm excited for my future. I'm happier now than I've ever been in my entire life. That's come from my wife, the support I've built up, and therapy. The problem for me is, I shouldn't have had to go through 20 years of torture and nightmares to get to therapy. I shouldn't have been mistreated just because I'm trans and queer.

Katy: Now that you've had some time to reflect on life – what achievements are you most proud of?

Lucy: So far, one of the things I'm most proud of in myself is that I am still open. As you know, I have gone through significant levels of trauma. My heart has been horrendously damaged. But one of the things I've held on to that is the crux of my personality – that one central thing that I hold on to – has been that I won't close my heart off. I will always try and see the best in people. I will always try and be the best I can be. I will always open myself up to love, and to hurt, because to do otherwise closes you off from who we are as humans at the most basic level. We are a species that thrives on community and needs connection.

If there's anyone who's reading this who feels like they can't do it, take heart – I have been through hell and back and I have found my nirvana. It is possible, whatever comes your way. Always try to hold true to who you are, and to keep your heart open. Even if it feels like your community is hidden in the shadows, we're out here for you.

Katy's post-interview thoughts

Although none of this was an infrequent topic of conversation between Lucy and me, I found that I left this interview with, somehow, a renewed sense of both hope and cynicism. Lucy's resilience and openness was a not exactly optimistic, but at least hopeful reminder that healing is possible, especially with help.

The conversation also serves as another reminder to research your mental health help well, if that's accessible to you. It's always okay to reach out for help, but it's prudent to be mindful of the kind of helper you might need. You definitely don't need or deserve the services of any mental health worker who is trying to steer you further away from who you really are. I wish that this was not something I had to recommend.

I also wish there was more support for people with profound lived experience of mental illness and neurodiversity to access therapy training. As discussed in my interviews with Sage, LJ, and Rory earlier in this book, therapy training is so often inaccessible to the people who could really make a difference, and this needs to change at all levels.

I miss Lucy endlessly and I'm glad that her caring nature, fierce love for her community, and inextinguishable sense of humour can be with you here. She continues to be a beacon of light in her community and she continues to make me proud every day.

If you'd like to know more

Samaritans. Lucy volunteered as a helpline operative with the Samaritans. If you're in the UK, you can contact them for mental health support by calling 116 123 or emailing jo@samaritans.org

LGBT Foundation. Lucy's recommendation for a helpful UK-based

LGBTQ+-focused support line was the LGBT Foundation. You can call them at 03453 303030 and email them at helpline@lgbt. foundation for support.

The Trevor Project. If you're looking for a North American option for LGBTQ+ mental health support, you can contact the Trevor Project by calling 1-866-488-7386 or using the chat feature at www. thetrevorproject.org/get-help

Pink Therapy. Pink Therapy offers a place to find vetted LGBTQ+-knowledgeable mental health practitioners. https://pinktherapy. com

Gendered Intelligence. Gendered Intelligence is a mental health directory for trans and gender-questioning people who are looking for counselling and therapy. https://genderedintelligence.co.uk/services/69-therapists-and-counsellors-network-directory

Love as Mental Health Care with Kai and Sorel

An introduction to Kai and Sorel

Kai and Sorel are two non-binary people living together and loving each other in England. I met Kai (they/them) when we were both in our early 20s and we immediately clicked, becoming best friends over the last decade or so. Kai went on to meet Sorel (she/they/ze) when Kai was in their late 20s and I've adored watching them both fall in love with each other. I knew I wanted to speak to Kai and Sorel because of how much I see them working together to support each other, and how important all kinds of queer love are to so many of us in the LGBTQ+ community.

I believe firmly that queer love is a healing force in a world that so often tells us we are undeserving of care. Trans people, in particular, are often told that love will be impossible for them (Gallo, 2023), and many trans people struggle to come out due to this projected isolation (McElroy, 2022). In reality, I've seen trans people experience all of the kinds of love and relationships that cis people do and, arguably, more. Reflecting on these kinds of love and care with Kai and Sorel was a delight, full of deep thoughts and laughter.

Since this interview, both Kai and Sorel have come to deeper understandings of their genders: a few months of HRT (hormone replacement therapy) has helped Sorel to realize they're 'more demi-girl than not a girl' and is using she/her/they/them/ze/zir pronouns, while Kai has come to the awareness that they are non-binary and is using they/them/their pronouns. To reflect this, you'll find me using their current pronouns in my writing about the interview but leaving the interview as-is, because, as Kai put it, 'it was true at the time'. I always love seeing people experiment with pronouns and learn new things about their identities, so I love this for both of them and I can't wait to see what else changes and stays the same between us all in the future.

Kai and Sorel's interview

Sorel: Hello! I am Sorel. I'm a non-binary transfem, they/them/ze/zir. I am bisexual, and I don't know if I'm also asexual – I'm still working that out.

I went to university to study physics and became a massive Space nerd out of that. If I hadn't done that I would have gone and studied English literature, which is a weird combination of choices, but I'm happy with the combination. I'm a big fan of Space and literature, which is not a Trivial Pursuit category.

Katy: [Katy laughs] It should be!

Kai: The category could be 'Space literature'!

Sorel: Yes! Space literature. It's the best.

Kai: I'm Kai. I'm a trans guy; I use he/him pronouns. I'm technically asexual and panromantic, but I just say I'm queer because that's easier to explain and less mouthy. Do I have anything interesting about me?

Sorel: Yes!

Kai: What, though? I don't know.

Katy: You are very interesting.

Kai: I'm never good at knowing what's interesting about me, though! It's hard to pick things out and think about that.

I am a guinea pig parent. That's my favourite thing, and I am a bit obsessed with guinea pigs. I am an aspiring author/artist, but only aspiring.

Katy: I mean, do you write? Do you think about art and writing? I think that makes you an author and an artist already.

Kai: I have a series of books I want to write. I want to write LGBTQ+ romcom books, mainly because I'm so tired of all the queer books and films having sad endings. There aren't really many queer books – there's more now, but a lot of them tend to be 'adult'. That's fine, but I wish there was a bit more variety.

Sorel: You also write all the fanfiction that you tell me about and no one else! Sorry. I don't have to have officially said that.

Katy: There's no shame in that!

So, you're both different flavours of neurospicy. What have your experiences of that been like?

Kai: I have diagnoses of anxiety, depression, and OCD (obsessive compulsive disorder). I also have a diagnosis of EUPD, but I don't really like the wording of that. I preferred when they called it 'borderline' – 'emotionally unstable' is a bit too on the nose.

I was also diagnosed with autism last year, but it was sort of expected. I've always had a feeling about it. Even though I think it is valid to self-diagnose, it is nice to have a professional agree with me.

Katy: What do you think you got from that professional agreement?

Kai: I have a bit of impostor syndrome, but having a diagnosis helps when a professional is telling you, 'You do have autism, you're not just making this up for attention.' I do really think self-diagnosis is valid because, if it fits you, I don't see why it's a problem if you've not got a professional diagnosis. The diagnosis helps, but it wasn't the start of my understanding that I'm autistic.

Sorel: I agree. We've found recently that the waiting lists to get professionally diagnosed are huge. Formal diagnosis is not always accessible.

Kai: I'm only where I am with this because I got to see a private psychiatrist. Even so, my psychiatrist wrote a letter to my doctor asking them to make a referral to my local autism support services, and my doctor was like, 'No, because you have to be diagnosed through us, so he'll have to wait another five years on the waiting list for that.' On one hand, having a professional diagnosis is good because it's easier to get support, but then the actual support is not that accessible anyway, unless you can afford private care, and I can't. The NHS support is underfunded. I was lucky enough to get that diagnosis funded through other means, because I wouldn't have been able to pay for it at all. I think the psychiatrist who saw me charges into the thousands for private patients.

Katy: I've been looking into this recently, because my health care providers have suggested I seek professional ADHD and autism diagnoses. I'm staring down the barrel of the massive NHS waiting lists, and paying privately means spending thousands of pounds that I don't have.

Kai: What you should do is commit a crime. [Everyone laughs] Get the government to pay for it.

Katy: Which crime would you recommend?

Kai: Something that you can blame on autism but that isn't gonna get you sent to prison.

Katy: For the sake of this book, I will state for the record that we're all joking. [Everyone laughs]

Sorel: For me, I am self-diagnosed with ADHD. It really fits me. Everyone always says I'm ADHD, so it's less that I'm fully self-diagnosed, just that I haven't seen a professional about it.

Katy: I always say that I'm peer-diagnosed.

Sorel: Exactly. I also have a professional diagnosis of anxiety, which is fun. I am an anxious bean. [Sorel tries to look through some notes and gets a little lost in what they're doing.] What am I doing? Sorry, I'm confusing myself. This bit is going in the book, of course?

Kai: I'd say this fits your ADHD self-diagnosis validity.

Sorel: Now this is the impostor syndrome coming up saying, 'But no, you're not. So let's have a panic attack about it instead!'

I've definitely thought I might also be autistic. I don't know. I don't know if I'm not. I've got ADHD and there's a large overlap, and that's why it feels like maybe it is but maybe it's not. I think there's also maybe some weird, internalized autistiphobia going on, too?

Obviously I don't think autism is bad, but maybe part of me thinks I can't be autistic because that will be bad for me.

My brain is definitely odd. It's not as easy to reassure yourself that you're not just weird when you don't have those stereotypical autistic traits, like being really into trains or engineering.

Kai: The stereotype for autistic people is allocishet white guys, which can make it difficult to understand yourself as autistic when you're anything else.

Katy: That's a huge mood.

Sorel: It's interesting, though, because I am a neurodivergent person who likes trains and engineering, just not to the same degree as other autistic people who are really, really fascinated by that. It feels different.

Kai: There is definitely a lot of overlap between autism and ADHD. I think that can make figuring this stuff out more complicated.

Katy: The research right now is kind of confusing, and there's a lot of overlap of traits. The stats show that most people with ADHD are also autistic, but it doesn't necessarily work the other way around, which is really interesting to me.

Sorel: That is interesting!

Katy: I also really hear you that it's an interesting experience when you think you might be autistic, but the way in which you experience your autistic traits is very different to the way in which autistic people are 'supposed' to show up.

Maybe I'm a good example, here. When I studied autism during my psychology degree, they taught us that autistic people don't experience empathy or have a theory of mind. That's obviously not true, but that was what I was taught 15 years ago. I spent ages being like, 'I have so many of these autistic traits, but I definitely can't be autistic because I have a lot of empathy. Sometimes too much empathy, in fact! I have so much empathy for people that it hurts. Sometimes I also feel really strongly for inanimate items and fictional characters, too.' And then, about five years ago, I discovered that hyper-empathy is an autistic trait, and I was like, [pleasantly surprised] 'Oh!'

Sorel: I've had almost that exact thing, to be honest!

Kai: I think it doesn't help that a lot of the research was done on allocishet white teenage boys. That's a specific group with quite a particular culture. I think people who aren't like that have often been missed in research. I don't know the actual stats, but I know girls and women with autism are massively underdiagnosed because they often present differently. Autistic people who are trans might add further confusion into that for researchers.

Katy: How did you both arrive at an understanding of your own genders and queerness, individually?

Sorel: My story is sort of long and meandering. I wouldn't say I'm one of the people who's always known from when I was a child, but I do remember that, as a child, as long as there's been an option while playing, I would choose the 'girl' option. I would play with the April O'Neil figure in my Ninja Turtles set. In *Golden Axe* I would play as the woman. In *Streets of Rage* I would play as the woman. In the little stories I wrote, they were always about women. So, going back, there's definitely a history of being more interested in femme people and identities.

I think the first time I really thought about it a bit more was in my teen years. When I was mid-teens – and probably before then, to be fair – it was a really 'hilarious' joke that boys made to say, 'I'm a lesbian trapped in a man's body' while leering at the girls, being sexist pigs. And I'd be like, '[sarcastically] Yeah, great, guys, well done. [brightly] Anyway, that really resonates with me for some reason that I'm not gonna think about.' I'd think about that phrase but not as a joke. At the time, I thought of myself as straight. In Facebook Memories, sometimes posts will come up where I was like, 'I'm a straight ally!' [Everyone laughs]

Then, in my mid-20s, which was the late noughties, I played an online game called *EVE Online*. Again, I chose to play as a girl character, as you do when you're very cis! Obviously, cis guys can, but I think they don't exclusively. I was finding myself yearning for something like a *Matrix* situation where I could meet in real life with the people I'd met through the game, and we could get together, and it wouldn't be like, 'Hey, you're a boy!' I wanted to spend time in the real world and be seen as the girl I was in the game.

Katy: It's so interesting, because I have heard this so many times! Even down to it being *EVE Online*, this is a really transfem experience!

Sorel: I'm not surprised. *EVE Online* is weirdly popular for trans people, I guess also because trans people love all the Space stuff? The ships are pretty cool, even though it is basically *Excel* the game.

I am an atheist and I was part of that New Atheism movement, as far as that was a coherent thing. I sort of retreated from other online environments while I was heavily playing *EVE Online*, and when I came back I sadly found my nice, rational, sensible, sceptical online society in a civil war over the idea that women aren't objects who should be treated like things. A friend of mine, who was very sensible and rational and whose opinions I had respected, was like, 'Glad to see you again. Have you heard of men's rights? Let's look into how feminism is cancer.' And I did, and I found out that feminism is, in fact, not cancer; it is actually quite cool and massively relevant.

Before then, I had thought that feminism was really important in the 1970s, and then women got the vote, and then everything for women was fine. [Sarcastically] Because I was really well educated! You know, I'd thought it was done. I had that white and 'generally seen as male' view on social issues back then. I was able to do my own research and found that, actually, things are not really that much better, and much improvement is needed. As part of that, I got involved in an online feminist group. One of the first things someone asked me was, 'What are your pronouns?' I defaulted to he/him because I'd never been asked that before. I was aware that trans people were a thing, and I was also aware that I was definitely doing a bit of a trans thing by kind of wanting to be seen as a girl, but also that didn't quite fit with me. I didn't really understand the question, so I went away and read about what they were asking me.

I did that reading and I found a blog which, stereotypically, might have been on Tumblr. The blog was someone talking about their experience of being non-binary. Well, I think it was 'gender-queer' at the time, because the term 'non-binary' hadn't been given social prominence at the time.

Katy: Genderqueer was definitely the word in the 2000s. That's what I first came out as, gender-wise.

Sorel: Yeah! So, reading that, I was like... There's a GIF that perfectly encapsulates this. It's a cat, and someone puts a little pink flower on its head, and it sort of pulls back, and then it's like the environment around it fades to black and then it's the warp effect, like the cat is going into lightspeed. That perfectly encapsulates that sort of 'Holy shit' feeling – like, 'Holy shit, this person is talking about me!' You know, this is full-on 'strumming my face with his fingers' shit, and I was just like, 'Holy shit, I'm genderqueer!'

So then I was like, 'I guess I'm a they/them!' And then like, three minutes after that – or maybe, like, a couple of months – I thought, 'And I'm probably bi.' Before, I had defined myself as 'straight-ish and boy-shaped', which is, again, definitely how straight cis guys think about themselves! [Everyone laughs]

So, that's basically my journey. At some point, non-binary became a more common term than genderqueer, and I went with that, although, to be fair, I still prefer genderqueer. It's a cooler term. But then cool doesn't really matter, I guess?

Katy: I think 'cool' can matter when it comes to gender! It's okay to want your gender to be cool! [Katy and Sorel laugh] That's gender euphoria right there.

Sorel: I prefer the non-binary flag, though, that's the thing! And the bi flag is prettier than the pan flag, which is part of why I say I'm bi!

Katy: They're good flags!

Kai: With me, I'll start with the sexuality side, because that was how it happened in real life. When I was in maybe Year 8, I remember thinking that I might have been bi. At the time, the way people talked about it back then, you were either gay, straight, or bi – those were the only options. As I got a bit older I realized cishet guys don't really do anything for me, so I thought maybe I was a lesbian. Then, one of my lesbian friends was like, 'Look at Shakira's newest music video!', and she was basically salivating over it, and I was like, 'Yeah, she's pretty, but I just don't get that.' I could appreciate someone's face, and then the body was just sort of there. I thought I was broken. I was like, 'Maybe I just don't feel sexual attraction like that? That can't be normal.'

I googled it, and it was a lot like Sorel said – when you find people who have the same experiences as you, and you find there's a word for it, that changes so much. That was how I found out about asexuality. It just resonated with me. I knew I wasn't aromantic, and I think that's why panromantic sort of fits me, because I've always found it possible to fall in love with anyone, regardless of their gender. So I accepted that in my early 20s.

The gender stuff was a bit more complicated. What I find quite funny is that, when I look back, I definitely see these signs that I was trans. I always related to boys in stories. As a child, I remember really connecting with *Mulan*.

Katy: A classic! [Kai and Katy laugh]

Kai: When she was like, 'Yes, I'm going to try to help my father by pretending to be a boy,' I was like, 'Wow, this story just speaks to me for some reason!'

When I was 12 or 13, my step-grandma used to love those really trashy 'life story' magazines. I remember I used to read them obsessively, and one of them had a trans woman's story, and that was the first time I'd ever actually found out that people could be trans. And again, I was like, 'Wow, something about this speaks to me, but I'm not sure what, so I'm just gonna pack that away fully.'

Later, when I was about 16 or 17, I said to my parents that I thought I was a boy, and I got a really negative reaction. I decided to just shove that back down and ignore it, which wasn't the best thing to do. I overcompensated for a while, and sometimes I tried to be super feminine while trying to tell myself, 'No, I am a girl!'

And then, once again, I learned that being non-binary was a thing. I was like, 'Well, maybe that fits me even better.' I was overcompensating so much, even to Sorel, and saying I was definitely still more on the feminine side, but something about that still seemed wrong.

One day, I was just sort of thinking about it all, and I was like, 'No. I am a man.' It just came to me. Luckily, Sorel was immediately accepting and supportive of it.

Katy: How did you two meet?

Kai: We basically matched on three different dating apps. I remember thinking, the first time I saw Sorel – which I think was on a Tinder – 'I've got a really good vibe about this person, and I really want to match with them.'

Katy: That's so nice!

Sorel: [Tearing up a little] I'm just here speechless!

Katy: It's okay! That's very cute. Do you think that being in a relationship together has changed how you think about gender and queerness?

Sorel: I think it has, for me. Before I met Kai, I was like, 'I'm definitely non-binary. I am definitely not a woman.' And like, I think I'm still...I still wouldn't... [Sorel takes a moment to think] I don't think I'm a trans woman in denial. But, again, I'm not sure. Right now I'm Definitely Not A Woman*. I mean, I'm definitely transfem, and that is something I thought before we were together, but it's something I thought quietly to myself and never where anyone else might hear it. Kai has changed that.

I've also changed my presentation. Before, I would occasionally wear a skirt at home when everyone else had gone to bed, when I was sat up playing on my computer at 2 am, like any healthy, normal, late-20s person. [Everyone laughs] Now, living with Kai, I'm sat in a nice, feminine top and a skirt right now, and I'm very comfortable. I could have never sat around like this previously. Being with Kai helps my ability to express myself more freely. Being able to actually express myself, and sit in my gender rather than keeping it hidden, has made this something I can be more certain about. This is actually me, being given the freedom to just live. Transphobes are like,

'Oh, it's just a costume,' and it's not. It's me, being myself, and being loved for being myself.

Katy: I feel there's something that's both so freeing and so grounding about just being able to be fully who you are with another person who loves you. I'm really glad that's something that you can have.

Kai: I feel similarly. Like I said before, my parents were really negative when I first came out. Having Sorel's full support helped me to be myself. Sorel didn't treat me any differently – I mean, obviously they treat me somewhat differently, but in the way I want. They still treat me like the same person I've always been. They immediately used my correct name and pronouns. They never treated me like I'm a weird freak just because I came out as a trans guy.

Neither of us are cis or het, so our relationship is definitely a queer one, but how that queerness is perceived by others has changed over time. When I used to present more femme we'd hold hands in public, but now, because I think we're both perceived as masc – even though Sorel's not at all masc – I'm afraid of being more affectionate in public. I'm scared of getting abuse from people for 'looking queer'. When Sorel is able to physically transition, and be read as femme, we'll maybe be read as straight, even though we're definitely not.

No matter how others see us, I've got a deeper understanding of my sexuality and gender just from having Sorel around. Having space with someone that allows you to be who you are has been really important.

Katy: What kind of support do you find most helpful to give the other partner, and to receive from the other partner?

Kai: I think, for me, emotional support is the most important kind of support, both giving and receiving. Especially with my mental health stuff, I like a lot of calm validation. I have had a lot of trouble with that in the past. I just thought I was sort of having tantrums, but it turns out I've been having autistic meltdowns. Sorel is always calm and supportive. It's helpful having someone who doesn't treat me like a monster for that. I've never been violent to Sorel, and I never would be, but I can be violent towards myself, or I'll hit objects just because I'm so frustrated and I need to let the energy out somewhere. I always feel bad, because obviously I know it can be scary to witness, but it does mean a lot having Sorel being a calm person with me.

Sorel: I know that meltdowns aren't Kai treating me badly; this is him having a really hard time. The way to deal with him having a hard time is not to treat it like it's something being done to me, like Kai is malicious and horrible, because that's not true. I don't hold anything against him. We can help each other get through it.

It helps to recognize where we both struggle. When my mental health is playing up, my thing is mostly just being totally silent. I guess that's selective mutism.

Kai: Can I add to that?

Sorel: Yes, of course.

Kai: Thank you. We've been together for about four and a half years and, when we were first together, when Sorel would go quiet, I used to be like, 'Oh, no, I've done something to upset them!' But now we know each other's reactions and triggers. I've learned what not to do, and I've learned how they like to be encouraged and cared for. I was careful to let them know that I wouldn't react badly to who they were, even if who they are in the moment is non-verbal.

Katy: It sounds like you can offer each other support without an expectation.

Sorel: It's such a huge thing, the difference that makes. It's healing just knowing how each other reacts, and that it isn't either of us being upset with the other or acting out maliciously, and knowing what might help. It's just the way we are when we're overwhelmed, and we know how to deal with it, how to support each other.

Katy: How do you work together towards good mental health for both of you?

Kai: We sort of do it naturally.

Sorel: We're just so mentally healthy! [Everyone laughs]

Kai: We're good at communicating with each other. I mean, there are some things we're not good at communicating, as well, but that's more individual stuff. There are some things, or certain moods I get in, where I don't want to bother anyone with my problems, but that's a 'me' thing, rather than a couple problem. As a couple, we do talk about things.

Katy: I think this type of care tends to come much more naturally when you like, respect, and love each other.

Kai: We're both also always trying to work on ourselves and our own well-being, and it's good to do that together. For example, I always had a lot of triggers around diet culture that I've worked hard to work through, and now Sorel works on them with me and in themself, too.

Katy: What do you think the future will be like for you two together?

Sorel: Hopefully it's good, and long, and full of guinea pigs.
I can feel both of us getting more emotionally resilient over time

from each other's support. That's how I feel, at least; I don't want to speak for you, Kai...

Kai: [Cheerfully] I think I'm always going to be a bit mental. [Katy and Sorel laugh]

Sorel: I think we all are. But I know we'll get each other through it.

Kai: Gender-wise, we both want to surgically transition eventually, in different ways. Obviously we're gonna need each other's support more than ever after that, for the recovery period. We both have that willingness to step in for each other when we can't do things. I think we'll have to go private, though. I know we'd need to save a lot, but it's probably still easier and quicker to save than to go on the waiting list for the NHS.

Katy: I imagine so, especially if you're looking at transmasc surgeries. I don't think there's anybody even doing phalloplasties on the NHS right now.

Kai: I'm not sure about bottom surgery because, even though I like the idea of the effects, the surgery and the recovery scares me. I definitely want top surgery.

Sorel: Speaking of the future generally, I have my fingers crossed that the current waiting list situation won't be like this in another ten years' time. I have hope that things will change. The current times that we're living in, it feels a lot like the late 1990s, early 2000s again, when there was so much pushback for being gay. There was this level of nonsensical obsession and opposition to gay people and marriage equality, and obviously it didn't just end overnight, but it got better. There was a time in my life when the hatred was constant, and it was painful to live in the same world as that. We now live in the time after that, where it's not perfect for gay people but it's been getting better. I'm hopeful that we're a couple of years from that with the transphobia in politics. It's horrible right now, and things are moving backwards, but it can't last.

Kai: I've seen that moral panics do have an end, when people realize that all the horror stories that are being threatened aren't actually happening.

Sorel: They'll realize that lesbians didn't go extinct! People are gonna see that the numbers of trans people aren't actually increasing exponentially. We aren't a sign of societal collapse. That level of fear and hatred just isn't sustainable. Things are definitely in the 'getting worse before they get better' phase, but I think it is gonna get better, and maybe we'll be able to get everything we want and need from the NHS without discrimination and with a reasonable wait, if the NHS still exists then.

Katy: It's always darkest before the dawn, right?

Kai: I'm less hopeful, more cynical, but of course I would like a world where it's better for people.

Sorel: To be fair, I have been called a sickly sweet, intolerable optimist in the past.

Kai: There's nothing wrong with being an optimist.

Katy: I'm glad that you're still an optimist.

Sorel: I can't help it. They can't take that from me. They haven't managed to beat it out of me.

Kai: We all grew up during Section 28, and we're still queer and trans. Trying to hide this from us, and take it from us – it didn't actually work. Queer and trans people aren't going to go anywhere, no matter how difficult they try and make it. There is a lot of pushback against this queerphobic moral panic. I do think we've got people on our side, and I am hopeful that, in the future, we'll be able to silence all the transphobia eventually.

Katy's post-interview thoughts

It's so interesting to me that, as we discussed loving and living as non-binary millennials, we ended up talking very closely about our neuroqueer experiences, especially in terms of our experiences as autistic, anxious, and ADHD queer folk. Sorel and Kai have worked on accepting each other's inward and outward experiences of neurodivergence with a willingness to step forward to help and an assumption that any hurt caused isn't on purpose. It's clear this has contributed a lot of trust and care to their relationship, and I've seen the importance of that consistent mutual care in all kinds of queer relationships, from care cooperatives in the community, to therapeutic work, to my own romantic relationship. Being willing to learn what each other needs, and to keep trying to show up to give each other that, is an important kind of love for all of us to give and receive.

If you'd like to know more

Trans Love: An Anthology of Transgender and Non-Binary Voices, edited by Freiya Benson, 2019. This book offers a selection of stories about all kinds of different love from all kinds of different trans and/or non-binary people. It's a rich and lovely exploration of how it feels to experience love as a trans person.

Twenty-Eight: Stories from the Section 28 Generation, edited by Kestral Gaian, 2023. Kai mentions in the interview that the three of us grew up under Section 28, which was a government act in the UK that made it illegal for LGBTQ+ lives to be discussed in schools from 1988 to 2003. This fantastic book explores the lasting impact of Section 28, and the damage that comes with isolating and demonizing the queer community.

Song of Achilles, by Madeline Miller, 2011. I asked Kai and Sorel what their favourite queer love stories were, and this was a big recommendation from Kai. It's one of my favourite books, too, but you'll need your tissues ready for the end.

Star Trek. More or less the entire *Star Trek* franchise, by Gene Roddenberry *et al.*, from 1966 to the present. While chatting about LGBTQ+ love stories, all of us agreed that *Star Trek* is pretty queer, from Kirk and Spock's longing looks at each other in the original series, to Garak flirting with Bashir over lunch in *Deep Space 9*, to the canon romance between Adira and Gray in *Discovery*.

Trans Joy with Stef Sanjati

An introduction to Stef

Stef Sanjati (she/her) is a Canadian neurodiversity and transgender advocacy expert, beauty content creator, and video game streamer. At the time of this interview, she was also the head narrative designer with Paidia Gaming. She's a woman with many hats to wear, and – as a queer trans woman with ADHD and Waardenburg syndrome – her work explores new ways to bring her audience accessible empowerment and joy. I've followed Stef's content over many years and through several different vibes, including her makeup tutorials, her deep dives into trans-affirming surgeries, her travel vlogs, her educational content, and her comedy sketches. I wrote a significant chunk of *The Trans Guide to Mental Health and Well-Being* while watching her gaming streams on Twitch, because the community she made on Twitch was so comfy!

Her recent focus on the things that bring her joy has been heart-warming to see. The concept of trans joy has meant a lot of things to a lot of people, from gender euphoria, to finding love and family in the trans community, to being at ease with yourself in daily life, to performing drag, and so much more. I know that some of the things that bring me trans joy are getting my undercut buzzed, when strangers use they/them pronouns for me without being told, and feeling connected to my body when I'm out in nature. This kind of joy is rarely part of the expected narrative around trans people (Siegel, 2023) but it's so important to recognize – and to feel. A lot of Stef's joy right now comes from beauty, gaming, stories, and her community, all of which I was delighted to explore with her in this interview.

I met with Stef for her interview at 10 pm my time and, though I was excited for our interview, I wasn't feeling particularly joyful. My hair was past due a cut and colour, and I felt scruffy and nervous, plus a little intimidated. I've been a long-time fan of Stef's content, and she always seems 'put together' in both her looks and her presence. I wasn't worried that she would judge me – she's much too kind – but knowing we were going to talk about the joy that beauty can bring trans people, while not feeling very beautiful myself, made me judge myself a little. I had to reassure myself that beauty means so many different things before we spoke, knowing that Stef would agree.

Stef's interview

Stef: I'm Stephanie. Online, I go by Stef Sanjati. My pronouns are she/her.

I've been a content creator for, gosh, over ten years. I started when I was 12 or 13 on Facebook and the OG (original) YouTube, doing makeup videos and the equivalent of shitposts in video form. Then, I went to school for makeup artistry. I went to a programme where I learned everything from bridal and fashion makeup, to sculpting monsters and prosthetics for television and film. I thought that was what I really wanted to do, but I ended up getting some success on YouTube when I was really young, about 18.

Around then I ended up discovering that I was trans. I started documenting my transition online, which is where my content creation career really took off. I created a large body of work that was all focused on trans education and teaching people – both cis allies and trans people – that were learning about themselves and the transgender community.

Then, around the beginning of the COVID-19 pandemic, I realized there was a part of me that I wasn't nurturing, and that was the gamer side of me. I've always been a gamer, all my life, and that was really central to my general enjoyment of things, but also to my gender experience and learning about it, and learning about who I was. So, I pivoted to gaming content in 2020, with the help of my partner, who did all my tech and helped me get everything set up and get started. Now I've been working in gaming for four years, and I became a Twitch partner with an amazing supportive community that I love. I ended up working in the games industry with a women-led organization called Paidia Gaming that has a mission to make the gaming world a more inclusive and kinder place. I've learned a lot as a professional in that environment.

Also, I have a dog that I love. Her name is Miss Ma'am, and she's lying on my feet right now. I'm a big dog person – that's a fact. And I live in my Big House of Gaming! Well, it's not that big – it's big for me because I'm used to a studio apartment. It's a Pretty Standard Size House of Gaming, where I live with my partner, and we love creating things and gaming together. It's a fun life. I'm really enjoying where I'm at right now.

Katy: It sounds like you have big things coming up in your career!

Stef: I feel really in control, and I feel really empowered to create things that I really want to create. I feel lots of momentum. I'm working with some game studios on some projects, to do some coverage and some content for games that I really love. I'm developing partnerships with other brands to amplify the legitimacy and the value of the shows that I can put on Twitch. I'm putting a lot more emphasis on Twitch, actually. I hope that's exciting – I'm really excited about it.

Katy: It sounds exciting!

Stef: [Stef laughs] Awesome! I took some breaks from streaming on Twitch for a while, and I did some personal work that needed to be done, and I realized that I really do love streaming. I love putting on a show; I love being an entertainer, and that's something that I wasn't allowing myself to lean into. So, with what I've got coming ahead, it's really like I'm stepping into my power as a businesswoman, and as an entertainer, and I feel like I'm gonna be able to bring into reality exactly what I want to bring, and that's a very good feeling. Certainly in terms of working more closely with game studios and with beauty brands and things that I really value – that's what I really want to do. I hope to keep going for the opportunities that I want, instead of waiting for things to come to me.

Katy: It sounds like you're bringing empowerment to yourself and to your community.

Stef: That's what I want! I really, really want to move into that empowerment. As you're aware, having been in the streams, for a long time there was a lot of emphasis on cosiness, which is cool! That was so needed at the time when I started streaming in 2020, with the pandemic and with everything that was going on. That's where I was at, and that's what I wanted to share – and what I wanted to receive, really, which is why I shared it. But, where I'm at now is definitely a different energy – still, I hope, the same tone, because I certainly still feel like compassion is at the front of it. It's just that, now, I feel like there's an element of action that compassion can give in terms of pushing yourself to do hard things, and feeling good about that, and being rewarded by accomplishing that. That's reflective, certainly, of where I'm at in my personal life. It always is when you're a streamer – I think you can't really make a separation there, even if you try.

Katy: Streaming seems like a profession where you have to be congruent. Like, if you're going to have fun with it, you have to be grounded in yourself and bringing your own energy.

Stef: Yeah, you do. If you're having a hard time, it's hard to bring that energy, right? I was having a hard time, there, for a while! [Stef laughs] But I'm feeling much better. It's exciting to see this marked difference in what I can actually do for people, in my audience and in my business. It's really cool to see recovery in action.

Katy: What are your favourite queer narratives to create?

Stef: I want to create narratives of queer empowerment. LGBTQ people experience harassment in gaming spaces, generally. Historically, there's been a lot of very loud exclusion, even if we're not in the room, and that has sucked. That creates an atmosphere of fear for people, where they feel like they can't participate. I want my work to show that you can participate. There are places you're welcome in if you want to do it, when you're ready. The narrative I want to show is that you can do it, and will be worth it. You can feel good about joining in, and you deserve to be here.

What I found in my personal experience – and certainly I come from a place of privilege within the trans community – is that I've been received far more respectfully in gaming spaces than I ever would have expected. A large part of what was holding me back was a learned fear from previous experiences, but time has passed. It's been a decade since I came out as trans. For a long time, I was still operating like it was 2014, and it's hard to realize that the world has actually changed. I had to think to myself, 'I don't have to be this anxious. How do I make that happen?' I like that narrative of seeing that things have changed, stepping into that, and saying, 'Okay, I want to change this even more. I want to feel better, and I can do something about that. What can I do?'

Katy: Do those narratives of empowerment cross over into your work with Paidia?

Stef: You can see that in my work with Paidia, too, which is where I get to do the games writing I always wanted to do. My job is to build a world, and create a fiction and characters for that world. That has been really fulfilling!

The primary protagonist of the world is named Mae, and she's actually named after Mae Jemison, the first Black woman astronaut – an incredible trailblazer. I adore her. Mae is a character who's a fish out of water in her Earthly life. She doesn't really fit in. She feels misunderstood by most people. She's in an academic setting and she's really interested in the subject matter, but she's not interested in the politics of how to actually get the research done, and how you have to speak and behave to navigate that environment. She ends up tumbling into this world of Paidia, which is a sci-fi fantasy world, across a dimensional portal. She finds herself feeling a lot more at home in this other world, and being able to be herself and contribute with her unique perspective and skills. She meets a woman there named Laurelei. We haven't developed a product where the story takes place yet, but this is 100% canon in the world of Paidia – those two characters end up falling in love and being together.

Certainly, Mae stumbles into another world by accident, but it's the idea that you can find your place where you feel good, where you feel empowered, where you're supported, where you're loved. I think that's an empowerment narrative as well.

Katy: How do you think your neurodivergence and your mental health experiences have influenced your creativity?

Stef: I have had a very rocky relationship with mental health. When I was younger, in my early 20s, I would have told you that my suffering made me a more creative person, and made me a more just person, and a more righteous person. What I've learned over the last few years – which has been part of my rough times and energy issues – has been that that is not the case. The suffering and the mental health issues that I've experienced have not made me a better artist. They have not made me a better person. They have been obstacles, and I've justified that in the past, especially creatively.

I used to really lean into making creative work about trauma. I think that can be really insightful and interesting, but the way that I was doing it as a creative person early in my content creation career, was I just kept opening wounds over, and over, and over. I just kept them open, and I kept airing them out, being like, 'Look at this wound!' Unfortunately, that was not creatively inspiring. I hit a wall. I thought that was all I had – that's what I believed, and the reality is that's not all I had, but it's all I was allowing myself to see. There's a narrative out there that being a struggling artist makes your art better. I think that's a really dangerous idea to indulge. I think that struggling can build character, but that doesn't mean that we need to. There's always a lesson to learn from struggling or suffering, but staying in it is not the desired outcome.

When it comes to neurodiversity I have a different opinion, because I don't think that's necessarily a negative experience. I think that's just a neurological born-in difference. When it comes to neurodiversity, I don't like to pathologize it as much. I can see, as a person that has ADHD, that I struggle regulating my attention, but I also see how that can help me creatively. My ADHD helps me to not get stuck in a plan, to be able to flex it and improvise. Certainly, I think it helps me with my speaking and on stream. I think that, interpersonally, it's important to think before you speak, and that's something I've had to learn! But creatively, I think being able to improvise what I'm saying on the go, as an entertainer, is a really helpful skill.

So pathologizing it all is a mistake, but saying it's a superpower and it's all good, that's also a mistake. I think it's just a difference, and there's things that you have to learn to accommodate for yourself. That's something I've had to really do – something even as simple as, for me, wearing the right kind of headphones that block out environmental noise. Or making sure that my dog is tended to before I sit down to focus on something, so she doesn't distract me, because I won't be able to get back on task. Or if there's daylight and I really need to focus on something, covering the windows so I don't get distracted by the outside world. It's those kinds of things. These are all little things, but these little accommodations, if I do all of them, I'm gonna see a lot more juice. I get a lot more out of what I can do if I notice what I need and I make that accommodation. Looking after myself in that way helps me be creative.

Katy: It's so important to let your creativity be accessible to you.

Stef: And to let it flow naturally. If I tried to say to myself, 'I have this great idea, but I can't give that attention right now, I have to focus on this outreach, or pitch, or whatever...' I'm going to still think about that idea, and I'm not going to do a good job at what I'm doing, because I'm refusing to let myself breathe in that area. So, what I do instead is, I'll write it down. I've ended up making a Discord channel for my business where I have different text channels for every project. So, if I have an idea, I just slam it into the brainstorming channel and then I can let it go. But not taking that five seconds or five minutes to let the idea breathe and put it somewhere – that is not accommodating myself, right? So, notepads, notebooks, Discord; those kinds of things are super helpful for me.

Katy: I might have to try a Discord channel, because I've been mostly using the Notes app in my phone, and then I look at that later, and...

Stef: ...And it doesn't make sense, right? Yeah, I've got a notebook here that's colour-coded text – everything colour-coding really helps me. But even this – like, I'll write something, and then I'll turn the page to go to another day, and I won't remember to look at that note again. I've found a lot of success with Discord – I've been really surprised. It's new for me this month, but I've been really thrilled with it.

Katy: How has your content changed as your body image has changed over the years?

Stef: So, like I said, I started content creation when I was 12 or 13. At that time I had a horrible relationship with my body image, but I didn't know what was going on. I was so young! I was still being really creative with makeup, and I was putting a lot of focus there, and that was really actually quite good. That was a healthy outlet for experimenting with my look and gender.

When I came out as trans, and I started documenting that, I was very vulnerable, and my content reflected that vulnerability. I certainly was a gentle and open person at the time, but I covered myself a lot, and I hid a lot – I would be very specific about lighting, and angles, and makeup, because I didn't want to be seen the way that I saw myself. That's rough to think about, because ultimately we should see ourselves in a positive light. Even if we're not 100% comfortable with everything physically, we still deserve to see ourselves as good. There are a lot of dangerous emotional connections we can make between our appearance and our confidence. When I was early in my transition I was experiencing a lot of dysphoria, but I still centred a sense of hope and progress. My content was about how I was going to work towards this gender affirming care, and how I was doing on hormones.

A bit further into my career, I got mixed up with some people that weren't the best influences on me. I started pushing things a little far. In terms of the trans community online, and especially trans women on YouTube at the time, there was a lot of pressure to look a certain way and to look really put together in a very specific way. You had to have the right lips, you had to have the right face shape and body, you had to have the extensions or wigs, and it had to all be super feminine and super socialite. I tried to resist that as best I could, but things got rough for me, and I started caving. Beauty stopped being about my empowerment and started being about comparison.

There was a time period where I was documenting body surgeries I was having, and I shared a lot of what was happening very explicitly, and I didn't think about it very much at the time. In hindsight, it started to get to a place where I really should have thought more about this. Speaking of the neurodiversity element, right? Impulse control with ADHD is rough! I didn't often think very far ahead. I was just like, 'This is going to be shocking and impressive.' Unfortunately, when you lean into shocking and impressive content and your body image is wrapped up in that, that gets very messy.

Ultimately that led to me withdrawing, because my body was telling me that something was not right. I was not healthy. I ended up going into a hospital programme for treatment for body image-related issues. That was complicated. I thought it was successful, and it was in that I don't have the image issues that I used to, but I also learned some other things in there that weren't so helpful. Once you get into that hard spot, it's hard to navigate into a really sound and secure way again. I think I'm there now, but it took a long time.

Then I pivoted to gaming when COVID happened. I wanted so much for the emphasis on my content to be about 'not me'. I used to be so particular about that, like, 'The audience can't be coming for me. They have to be coming for the show.' I think, in doing that, I was doing myself a bit of a disservice. Underneath that, there was this idea that I'm not worth it for people to come to see me. I stopped taking care of myself, because I didn't feel like I was worthy of it. That's something that I have worked really hard to fix, from a mental wellness perspective first and foremost. That self-care has involved a lot of hard lessons, and a lot of action that I never thought I would have to take about different things in my life. That's what landed me in this place now, of empowerment.

Now, my content isn't really about my body image. It can be about my transness, to an extent – certainly, I want to bring trans people in, and I want to create space for them. I can do that as a visible trans person, by saying I'm trans online, by putting the trans tag on my streams, by talking about it and doing advocacy work. Part of that is still rooted in my love for beauty, and that is a tool that I want to use to empower people – not just to empower myself, although I certainly love to empower myself with it – but I want to show people that you can be creative with it. You can be fun with it. I recently did a *Halo* makeup look, and I took a photo with a Master Chief helmet, and I posted saying the game *Halo* was for everyone standing in the face of transphobia. Makeup is part of that. It's not just the words.

I feel empowered in my body image now, and that's coming through in my content, but it's been a rocky road over a decade of figuring that out.

Katy: It sounds like, right now, there's that element of what we were saying earlier – about standing in your energy. About being able to express your body, your image, and your self, in a way that means you can play and have fun with who you are. That's so important!

Stef: I love being able to embody the spirit of play! Life should feel good! I think that's easy to lose sight of – that life should be fun. Now I know that, when things don't feel good, it's my responsibility to ask for help. I have community; I have people that love me. If I'm struggling, I need to ask for help, and use my voice.

Katy: What helps you to connect and be grounded?

Stef: This is new for me, but what's been working really well for me is meditation. I do the same five-minute guided meditation YouTube video. It's free. I lie down on my bed – I work from home, so I can do that – and I close my eyes, and I just let it go.

Letting go is something that I particularly needed help with. When it comes to being grounded and connected to your body, a big part of that is actually knowing how you feel. And then actually feeling it! Unfortunately, until maybe a year ago, I didn't know that emotions were physical feelings. I intellectualized everything I felt and thought non-stop, and I would justify feelings, and I would explain feelings, and I would do everything but feel them. What was really important, to connect and be grounded in my body, was letting myself feel these emotions, and then letting them pass. I would get so stuck in the feeling, and I'd be like, 'Is this just all I am anymore? Just angry? Or just ashamed, or just sad?' And then, instead of feeling that way, I would just say, 'No, I'm not.' But not feeling it meant it would stay. Now, I'm feeling it and letting it go through me. Then, I feel connected. I'm calm. I'm grounded.

There're also other care rituals, like doing my makeup and getting dressed. During the pandemic, I would wear sweatpants and a T-shirt. This is great, by the way – there's nothing wrong with this – but, for me, the problem was that it was every day for years. I wouldn't get dressed. I wouldn't do my hair. It's not that dressing this way felt good, but that it felt bad to try anything else. I was depressed, frankly. I wasn't taking good care of myself physically. A big part of that was not being connected to my body, not being grounded. When I don't do those care rituals, I don't check in with how I'm feeling.

So, doing those care rituals and checking in with myself helps – and, honestly, I still need reminders from my partner often. He'll gently tell me that I look stressed and ask if I need to go do a meditation. At one point I might have been like, 'No!' But now I try to say 'Okay, maybe I am. Thank you for offering that suggestion.' It's a tricky journey but, in making the time to feel feelings, you spend a lot less time being consumed by them.

Katy: I think that's such a common journey with neurodivergent people, and with people who have some kind of trauma. It can be so difficult to get the feeling out when you don't have access to the felt sense of it.

Stef: I have become aware that this is a pretty universal experience, and I'm grateful for that. Actually, it makes me feel connected to other people. I honestly wish for anybody that has that experience of not knowing how they feel in their body to have that journey. I think we all deserve to, and I'm really grateful that I was able to.

I give a lot of credit to my partner and my friends for consistently reminding me that I'm worth that, and pushing me in the right direction, because I don't know if I would have figured it out without people telling me that this is a problem. They wanted me to be okay. It took a long time, even with those reminders, so I am really grateful to the people in my life – and people in anyone's life – that are willing to stand with somebody and help them work through this. That takes a lot, and I have a lot of respect for that.

Katy: I'm so glad that you have such a kind community around you. What do you think makes for a healthy queer community?

Stef: The queer community is many things, including a community full of marginalized and traumatized people. It's really important for there to be awareness of triggers, and awareness of topics that might be harmful to hear. It's important to be mindful in a healthy queer community.

I also think it's important to have that element of strength, encouragement, and solidarity for everyone, in a way that isn't solidarity in fear. We can also have solidarity in the will to overcome, the will to persevere, the will to progress. Having our LGBTQ community around us is important, but we do a disservice to ourselves when we insulate our environments so intensely that we can't even see another one. When we isolate ourselves, our tolerance level for stress, or tolerance level for challenge, or tolerance level for anything, really – all of that goes down. I think that's where it gets messy, and this is where I've struggled recently with the 'cosy community' idea. It's good to close ranks, but then how do we then go out? Because we don't want to be stuck in the cave, right? I don't.

That's something that I am trying to think about a lot as I move into this more empowered phase of my content and my streaming. I'm thinking a lot about how I make space for people that need protection and care, and how I can also encourage those people to push their comfort zone at a healthy rate. I want my community to feel more secure, more valued, more empowered, more emotionally safe, so that they can then explore and have fun.

It is important to develop those skills of emotional capability and resilience, and that can be really hard, especially for neurodivergent people. ADHD affects emotional pain processing and reactivity, and I used to say, 'I can't fix that!' And I can't – it's not fixed, and it didn't need to be fixed – but I can still work with who I am to improve my reactions. I thought I couldn't control my impulses, but that wasn't true. It was really hard to get to a place where I could understand that, because I was getting a lot of feedback from people that my ADHD meant I couldn't control myself and I'd have to be okay with that. But we can change!

I hope we can keep each other safe and also empower each other to then go out into the world, and be strong, and capable, and make change, or even just live a happy life. We deserve to live without constant stress, without constant anxiety, without constant fear. As a queer person – as a trans person – what a gift it is to go through a day without stress!

When I say it's important to challenge your comfort zone, it's not to stress a person out. There are limits. What I want is to help queer people reduce their stress around the fun and important stuff. It's about creating healthy challenge with support and encouragement.

Katy: I hear you. It's about helping ourselves to be able to assess for danger, safety, and enjoyment, while calming our hypervigilance.

Stef: Yes! Yes, hypervigilant is the word. I used to just embody that. Trauma makes you think it's helpful, but that's not a healthy trait. It's hard to face that and acknowledge that you're operating all the time on this level of constant threat. 'What is that doing to me? What is that doing to the people around me? What's that doing to my dreams – to the things that I want to achieve?' Gosh, that's a hard conversation to have with yourself. Especially when you don't even know you have to have that conversation with yourself. You have to be brave.

Katy: I feel like your content creation has been really brave when you've looked at those tough moments in your life. It's also been really brave when you've put down firm boundaries around that and focused on trans joy. So, I'm wondering what trans joy means to you?

Stef: My understanding of that has evolved. Originally, I thought of trans joy as a gender euphoria thing – that when I feel beautiful, when I don't feel dysphoria, I feel trans joy. I still think that's a form of it.

Then it became about the moments when I don't even think about transness, and I get to just live a 'normal life'. It doesn't quite make sense to me now, but my idea at the time was that it's the privilege of living a life without having to think about this – that ideal was joyful. I think maybe that's what I needed at the time, but I don't think that's what I would tell people any more.

Now, I think what trans joy is, again, is stepping into our power.

Something I've done a lot of work on, personally, is to stop trying to forget that I'm trans, because that's a rejection of myself. Ultimately, I feel I am a trans woman. I always will be, and that's cool! There are unique things about that experience that are valuable and interesting, and that I should share with people. I used to hear statements like that and think it wasn't fair but, when I say I'm a trans woman and I always will be, it's not that that's anything worse than being a cis woman. Those are just two different experiences, and I have information, wisdom, and experience that a cis woman just won't have. My transness is a whole, valuable component of the self. To deny it means you're missing something for yourself. If I reject that, I reject myself. In that way, my trans joy is the joy of accepting.

There is power in accepting that I am trans, and also that I'm a businesswoman, and also I'm an entertainer, and also I'm a dog mom, and also I have this relationship, and also I love my friends. I'm trans in all of that. When I talk with my friends about gender, I'm trans. When I talk about anything else, I'm trans. I'm trans with my dog, you know? [Both laugh] It's not that I'm trans and I'm always happy. It's that I don't have to not be trans to be happy. I don't have to reject that to be happy. I don't have to hide that to be happy. Of course, different people in different situations are gonna have different levels of access to that reality. That's important to acknowledge. But for me, what is transforming to me, is that I can just be...me!

Honestly, just living a life that makes me happy while being trans is harder than it should be. For life to just be simple...that can be important to find. To feel safe, secure, and happy, and to feel like I'm accomplishing the things I want, just to live a fulfilling life while trans – that's hard to get. That's hard to achieve because of the world that we have come up in.

But, like I said earlier, ten years have passed since I came out, and things have changed. I moved back to my home county, which I said I would never ever, *ever* do, thinking that I would have some trouble with the locals. It turns out that the people in the community have been the least of my problems. They've actually been great. I've seen pride flags, and trans flags, and progress flags in the windows of businesses that I never would have seen growing up here.

One of my neighbours is a trans kid. I was the only trans kid in my neighbourhood, and seeing a trans kid around the age that I was when I started experiencing really hard things at school, it was huge to me. They're not experiencing that level of hatred. They have their own difficulties, but it's improved enough that this kid can actually be outside. They can ride their bike in the neighbourhood. They have friends. Being able to also be there for that kid, and to see them happy, that was a transformative experience. It was like talking to myself at that age – the parallels that still exist are significant, but they're happy. It was very fulfilling to be able to speak to somebody that's in the position that I was and see them doing better. The kids are gonna be all right! What I stood up for when I was here at that age has made a difference, because now this child does not have to suffer the same way. There's this concept that goes around of like, because I suffered, somebody else should have to as well. That often comes up in conversations about social equity or access to resources. I'm a firm believer that people should not have to suffer like I suffered, and that's trans joy, too – seeing younger trans people understand that they're trans at 13, instead of being confused and lost. Seeing a kid be able to understand that – oh my gosh, that's trans joy. Seeing the world get better, seeing the world understand us better, seeing kids be accepted by their families – oh my goodness, that's a communal trans joy. I think that's really special.

Katy: I love that phrasing – 'communal trans joy'. I'm so glad that kid gets to see your trans joy in being a trans adult, too.

Stef: I would have loved that as a kid! I take that really seriously. I'm grateful for the opportunity to provide that to them. I feel like I owe it to them.

Katy: What brings you trans joy most often?

Stef: Something just came to me really hard and strong there, and it's being present with my partner and my friends.

I always kept people at arm's length as a trans kid, because I had a lot of trouble with people staying my friend. Once I came out, people just started being weird with me, not wanting to be seen in public with me, things like that. It was hard. As an adult, even when I had friends, I still kept them at arm's length, and I didn't really understand what friendship should feel like or how to treat people. Unfortunately, that's the side effect of trauma that I think a lot of people, especially trauma survivors, don't like to talk about, because, unfortunately, this has made me be an arsehole before. I've struggled to talk about that because, honestly, I don't want to make other people feel uncomfortable, but I think it's really important to acknowledge.

Now, I feel joy being with my friends. I love hopping on a call with my partner and my friends, and playing a game together, and being able to laugh and relax and be myself, and not feel like I need to watch what I'm saying or how I'm behaving, not questioning if they really like me. That insecurity still comes up once in a while, but I can recognize it as an insecurity. I can trust these people. Feeling relaxed in friendship, oh my gosh, that is such a joy.

I remember a specific moment of trans joy when I realized, 'Oh, I have friends!' I was sitting there playing a game with my friends, and I realized consciously that I had friends, and that was just beautiful. Growing up as a trans kid, that wasn't something I always had, and something I didn't always know what to do with.

Being able to be present with that – to recognize that things are going well in my life, to recognize that I have a community that comes to these streams that I put on, to recognize that I have the professional respect of my peers in business, to recognize that I can reach out to a company that I really like and get an enthusiastic response, to realize that, hey, I'm a cool person, I deserve these things, I deserve for people to be kind to me, I deserve to be present. That brings trans joy.

Friendship is a powerful joy, maybe because that's the most powerful form of others' understanding. I can be relaxed around other people. I can trust people. It reminds me to be grateful, and to appreciate that, and to really care that that's happening.

Katy: I've seen some of that when you've been streaming the community gaming nights. Everybody seems so relaxed and happy to be with each other.

Stef: Oh, that's so cool! I'm so glad to hear that. That's definitely the energy that I wanted. That's so nice to hear that it's making me a little emo!

That's part of why I wanted to do the community gaming streams. Remember I was talking about the game *Halo*, and about queer people being afraid of being reacted to with hostility in games? For me, my anxiety with gaming spaces was also connected with that social anxiety that I picked up in my early friendships. When Travis (Stef's partner) first tried to get me to play *Halo*, I would break down in tears – I would get so overwhelmed and completely dissociated. It was awful. It was really hard. Being able to play that game with other queer people, with all queer friends – oh my goodness, I am so grateful for that. I knew it might be hard to get a big queer audience invested in watching me play FPSs (first-person shooters), which is why I was like, 'Okay, let's bring them in to the game!'

I want people to join if you've never played before, if you're anxious. This is why I'm doing the show. I want people to come and play, and see that this can be so relaxing and fun. Really, it's not just about the game; it's about what experiencing that game with friends is like. That experience was – and is – a huge part of me finally accepting that I can trust people.

Katy: It's just really... The word that's coming to me is 'nice'? That doesn't seem like a strong enough word.

Stef: I think that it is a strong enough word! 'Nice' can be a big deal. 'Nice' means that everything's good, that there's some positivity. It's awesome that it's nice! I think things should be nice more often.

Katy: How else have you found joy and empowerment in gaming?

Stef: When I was a kid, I started with top-down RPGs (role-playing games) and RTSs (real-time strategies) like *Diablo*, *Nox*, and *Warcraft II*. I loved them, but it wasn't really until I played *Diablo II*, and I could play as the Amazon and the Sorceress characters, that I was like, 'Ooh, something about this is cool!' When I would observe older boys and the way they interacted with those female characters, I could tell there was a different energy to it, and I would not feel that kind of energy when I looked at those characters – I didn't get it. I was just like, 'Oh, she looks so cool! Oh, look at her ponytail!' [Both laugh]

Then, *Warcraft III*: the Night Elves in their matriarchal society; Tyrande and her leadership; all these bad purple bitches just doing cool things! There was something about that that I really, really loved and resonated with. I always gravitated towards these feminine archetypes, roles, and characters in video games.

The game that I've played the most in my life has been *World of Warcraft*, and my first characters were men. There came a time when I started thinking, 'I want to play a girl character – what's wrong with that?' I would always encounter this idea that I shouldn't do that. When I was younger, I played with Barbie dolls, and I was given negative feedback from certain people – not my parents, but in general, like if I talked about it at school or whatever. So, the idea that I shouldn't do girl things was passed on to me, but I started playing female characters in private because, why not? That helped me see more that I liked it, that it was comfortable, that I wanted to lean into that. Then, I would slowly but surely get more and more comfortable choosing the feminine option in front of people. I would play *Morrowind* or *Oblivion* and make a female character. These games meant I could have these experiences, and they increased my confidence to do that.

I have this character that I play in *World of Warcraft* – it's my Blood Elf Rogue, name Layorin. She was once named Layz, and she was not a woman when I first made her, but I was able to change her gender. At the time you had to pay *Blizzard* to change your character's appearance and gender. You don't have to pay for that any more – you can just go to a barber shop and they can change your gender for free. Wouldn't that be great? But at the time, I was very intentional – I was going to change this character's gender so that I could feel comfortable playing her. Because I love this character! I made her when I was 11. I'm 28, and she's still my main character. I feel like I've gone on that journey with that character, and being able to mirror that somewhere was so important to me. Video games are such a safe environment to do that for kids, and for anybody.

I love the power that video games can have, whether that's challenging social anxiety on Halo Night with a community, or experimenting with gender in RPGs, or encountering a story about something political in a game and it changing your perspective a little bit. All of those things are way bigger than the game, and certainly when it comes to trans rights there's a lot of power there. I think, in general, video games as simulations – as experiences for us to process information in – can bring such power to every aspect of our life. I think we're gonna see a lot more research and information about that in the next couple of decades. I'm really excited to see what that is like, and I want to be a part of something that encourages that thought. I would like to continue encouraging people to use video games as an avenue for exploring themselves, for challenging themselves, for bettering themselves, and for living a happier and more healthy life. They don't have to just be an escape and a distraction. They can be a tool to improve the way you feel every day. Not just to avoid how you feel, but to improve how you feel.

Katy: God, this makes me think about when I was doing my BSc in psychology, and all of the research that we were given about video games was that they were bad for people.

Stef: [Sarcastically] Well, that's not biased…!

Katy: The research was always about how gaming made people violent and unfocused, that games made kids antisocial, that they'd give you ADHD – it's not even like ADHD is a bad thing, but also, that's not how any of this works!

Anyway, when I was done with my studies, psychological ideas around gaming were starting to change. Now – and particularly around the pandemic – I've seen so much mental health stuff involving gaming pop up. There are self-care apps like *Finch*, and therapy groups run in *Minecraft*, and co-op farms on *Stardew Valley* that are based around good mental health practices.

Stef: That's lovely! I think video games have a lot of power to help people stay well. This is completely speculation – I'm not a scientist – but I think video games can help us stay sharp, because they help us think about all these different skills, like strategy, coordination, communication, reading, all of that. There's so much to engage the mind. I think that we're going to see the application of video games in areas well beyond just enjoyment really soon. I think it's already starting, but I think there's so much room for that to grow. I'm excited for the future of it all. Knowing I'll be 90 and still playing video games – that brings me joy!

Katy's post-interview thoughts

Even though I probably left the interview scruffier and more tired looking than ever, my conversation with Stef helped me to connect with the beauty that comes with self-expression, friendship, confidence, and play. I'm so glad we got to end the last interview of this book with joy, because it's such a core part of the queer experience, even with everything stacked against us.

Since this interview I've been thinking a lot about Stef's bravery as a step towards joy. Exploring our optimal widow of tolerance (Siegel, 2010) in a gentle way can help us to decrease our hyper-vigilance (Krupnik, 2021) – which is to say, gently pushing yourself beyond your usual comfort zone in a kind and self-consensual way can help you to feel safer and more in control of your life. Doing this is about increasing your sense of joy and comfort, not about punishing yourself to do and be more, and there are loads of ways that this bravery can look. I would say that a lot of my brave joy over the last few years has been about properly assessing where my comfort zone even really is – I've been in the process of learning what it means to rest and be still, which has been so alien to me that slowing down and learning to be cosy has taken its own kind of bravery. Your own next brave little push will be entirely unique. What would you like to explore next?

If you'd like to know more

@stefsanjati on Twitch. Stef's gaming stream, where you can join the LGBTQ+-friendly community and watch Stef play a range of games, often with fantasy and sci-fi themes. www.twitch.tv/stefsanjati

Stef's YouTube channel. This is a place where you can learn more about beauty, well-being, gaming, and trans joy. www.youtube.com/@StefSanjatiOfficial

Paidia Gaming. Stef was the head narrative designer for Paidia Gaming, an inclusive and woman-led gaming community and tournament platform. https://paidiagaming.com

Gender Euphoria, edited by Laura Kate Dale, 2021. A collection of stories from trans, non-binary, and intersex writers regarding their experiences of gender euphoria and trans joy.

Last Thoughts on the Things that Help

While discussing mental health and neurodiversity with so many experts of so many kinds throughout this book, I've been honoured to be with each collaborator's uniqueness. It's also been exciting to notice a number of patterns emerge from their experiences of what has been helpful for the emotional, mental, and communal health of LGBTQ+ people. I want to leave you with some of our combined ideas about what might help you and your queer community going forward.

My queer mind loves lists, so I've collated some of my interviewees' wisdom into lists of short suggestions to think on, collected into three main categories: be yourself, be with others, and seek joy.

Be yourself. Be present with yourself and your needs. Be in your body. Embrace your unique queer insight. Check in with yourself. Ask yourself what you need. Aim for self-direction. Take the intersections of your experiences of oppression and privilege in to account. Rest.

Be with others. Find safe people like you. Find safe people who aren't like you. Hold space for each other. Learn what you need together. Practise empathy. Explore vulnerability. Seek mental health professionals with knowledge and lived experience of queerness, neurodivergence, and trauma. Engage in activism and community care. Understand that intersectionality across marginalization strengthens the queer community. Hold your pets tight (if they're into that). Trust that you can make a difference. Love in as many ways as possible.

Seek joy. Delight in your dreams. Present yourself to the world however feels right, whenever it feels safe to do so. Trust yourself. Hang on to hope and optimism. Play, create things, and have fun. Do what works for you, even if it's unusual. Get weird with it. Believe in queer magic. Be with however you're feeling, even if it's not joy right now. Cherish yourself and your queer mind.

References

Abbate-Daga, G., Amianto, F., Delsedime, N., De-Bacco, C., and Fassino, S. (2013). 'Resistance to treatment and change in anorexia nervosa: a clinical overview.' *BMC Psychiatry*, 13, 1.

Ashley, F. (2023). 'Interrogating gender-exploratory therapy.' *Perspectives of Psychological Science*, 18, 2, 472–481.

Berke, D.S., Maples-Keller, J.L., and Richards, P. (2016). 'LGBTQ perceptions of psychotherapy: a consensual qualitative analysis.' *Professional Psychology: Research and Practice*, 47, 6, 373–382.

Bizzeth, S.R. and Beagan, B.L. (2023). '"Ah, it's best not to mention that here": Experiences of LGBTQ+ health professionals in (heteronormative) workplaces in Canada.' *Frontiers of Sociology*, 8, 1138628.

Blakemore, E. (2023). 'Gay conversion therapy's disturbing 19th century origins.' *History*. www.history.com/news/gay-conversion-therapy-origins-19th-century.

Blosnich, J.R., Farmer, G.W., Lee, J.G., Silenzio, V.M.B., and Bowen, D.J. (2014). 'Health inequalities among sexual minority adults: evidence from ten U.S. states, 2010.' *American Journal of Preventative Medicine*, 46, 337–349.

Bruce, H., Munday, K., and Kapp, S.K. (2023). 'Exploring the experiences of autistic transgender and non-binary adults in seeking gender identity health care.' *Autism in Adulthood: Challenges and Management*, 5, 2, 191–203.

Burton, N. (2024). 'When homosexuality stopped being a mental disorder.' *Psychology Today*. www.psychologytoday.com/us/blog/hide-and-seek/201509/when-homosexuality-stopped-being-a-mental-disorder.

Butler, J. (1990). *Gender Trouble: Feminism and the Subversion of Identity.* New York: Routledge, Chapman and Hall.

Cai, H., Chen, P., Zhang, Q., Lam, M.I., *et al.* (2024). 'Global prevalence of major depressive disorder in LGBTQ+ samples: a systematic review and meta-analysis of epidemiological studies.' *Journal of Affective Disorders*, 360, 249–258.

Capaldi, M., Schatz, J., and Kavenagh, M. (2024). 'Child sexual abuse/exploitation and LGBTQI+ children: context, links, vulnerabilities, gaps, challenges and priorities.' *Child Protection and Practice*, 1, 100001.

Carrington, M. and Sims, M. (2024). 'How can counselling training courses better prepare their trainee therapists to work with LGBTQ+ clients?' *Counselling and Psychotherapy Research*, 24, 2, 513–523.

Chamlou, N. (2024). 'Diversity in the mental healthcare profession: then and now.' *Psychology.org.* www.psychology.org/resources/diversity-in-mental-healthcare.

Chan, A.S.W., Choong, A., Phang, K.C., Leung, L.M., Tang, P.M.K., and Yan, E. (2024). 'Societal discrimination and mental health among transgender athletes: a systematic review and meta-analysis.' *BMC Psychology*, 12, 1, 24.

Chen, J.H. and Shiu, C.S. (2017). 'Sexual orientation and sleep in the U.S.: a national profile.' *American Journal of Preventative Medicine*, 52, 433–442.

Connolly, M.D., Zervos, M.J., Barone, C.J., Johnson, C.C., and Joseph, C.L.M. (2016) 'The mental health of transgender youth: advances in understanding.' *Journal of Adolescent Health*, 59, 5, 489–495.

Cooper, K., Mandy, W., Russell, A., and Butler, C. (2023). 'Healthcare clinician perspectives on the intersection of autism and gender dysphoria.' *Autism*, 27, 1, 31–42.

Cooper, M., Mearns, D., Stiles, W.B., Warner, M., and Elliot, R. (2004). 'Developing self-pluralistic perspectives within the person-centered and experiential approaches: a round table dialogue.' *Person-Centered and Experiential Psychotherapies*, 3, 3, 176–191.

Davies, D. and Barker, M.J. (2015). 'Gender and sexuality diversity (GSD): respecting difference.' *The Psychotherapist*, 60, 16–17.

DeChants, J.P., Green, A.E., Price, M.N., and Davis, C.K. (2024). '"I get treated poorly in regular school – why add to it?": Transgender girls' experiences choosing to play or not play sports.' *Transgender Health*, 9, 1, 61–67.

De Pedro, K.T., Shim-Pelayo, H., and Bishop, C. (2019). 'Exploring physical, nonphysical, and discrimination-based victimization among transgender youth in California public schools.' *International Journal of Bullying Prevention*, 1, 218–226.

Dewinter, J., De Graaf, H., and Begeer, S. (2017). 'Sexual orientation, gender identity, and romantic relationships in adolescents and adults with autism spectrum disorder.' *Journal of Autism and Developmental Disorders*, 47, 9, 2927–2934.

Ellis, E. and Cooper, N. (2013). 'Silenced: the Black student experience.' *Therapy Today*, 24, 10.

Fadus, M., Hung, K., and Casoy, F. (2020). 'Care considerations for LGBTQ patients in acute psychiatric settings.' *Focus*, 18, 3.

Ferreira, L. (2024). 'New guidelines for schools "encourage discrimination" against trans students.' *Open Democracy*. www.opendemocracy.net/en/gender-questioning-children-consultation-respond-discrimination-trans-students.

Flores, A.R. (2021). 'Social acceptance of LGBTI people in 175 countries and locations: 1981 to 2020.' UCLA School of Law, Williams Institute. https://williamsinstitute.law.ucla.edu/publications/global-acceptance-index-lgbt.

Ford, Z. (2013). 'APA revises manual: being transgender is no longer a mental disorder.' *ThinkProgress*. https://archive.thinkprogress.org/apa-revises-manual-being-transgender-is-no-longer-a-mental-disorder-8b0321f775d2.

Formby, E. (2013). 'The impact of homophobic and transphobic bullying on education and employment: a European survey.' International Lesbian, Gay, Bisexual, Transgender and Queer Youth and Student Organisation/Sheffield Hallam University. https://shura.shu.ac.uk/10144/1/Formby_-_Bullying_Report_-_WEB.pdf.

Fortunato, A., Giovanardi, G., Innocenzi, E., Mirabella, M., *et al.* (2022). 'Is it autism? A critical commentary on the co-occurrence of gender dysphoria and autism spectrum disorder.' *Journal of Homosexuality*, 69, 7, 1204–1221.

Fredriksen-Goldsen, K.I., Kim, H.J., Barkan, S.E., Muraco, A., and Hoy-Ellis, C.P. (2013). 'Health disparities among lesbian, gay, and bisexual older adults: results from a population-based study.' *American Journal of Public Health*, 103, 1802–1809.

Freud, S. (1899). *The Interpretation of Dreams*, trans. 1913. London: Macmillan.

Gallardo-Nieto, E.M., Espinosa-Spínola, M., Ríos-González, O., and García-Yeste, C. (2021). 'Transphobic violence in educational centers: risk factors and consequences in the victims' wellbeing and health.' *Sustainability*, 13, 4, 1638.

Gallo, Z. (2023). 'Romance, intimacy and love while trans.' *Say It Out Loud*. https://sayitoutloud.org.au/learn-more/romance-intimacy-love-while-trans/?state=al.

George, R. and Stokes, M.A. (2018). 'A quantitative analysis of mental health among sexual and gender minority groups in ASD.' *Journal of Autism and Developmental Disorders*, 48, 6, 2052–2063.

Goffman, E. (1956). *The Presentation of Self in Everyday Life*. Edinburgh: Doubleday.

Goodier, M. (2023). 'Hate crimes against transgender people hit record high in England and Wales.' *The Guardian*, 5 October. www.theguardian.com/society/2023/oct/05/record-rise-hate-crimes-transgender-people-reported-england-and-wales.

Gorden, C., Hughes, C., Astbury-Ward, E.M., and Dubberley, S. (2017). 'A literature review of transgender people in prison: an "invisible" population in England and Wales.' *Prison Service Journal*, 233, 11–22.

Gordon, A.R., Austin, S.B., Pantalone, D.W., Baker, A.M., Eiduson, R., and Rogers, R. (2019). 'Appearance ideals and eating disorders risk among LGBTQ college students: the Being Ourselves Living in Diverse Bodies (BOLD) study.' *Journal of Adolescent Health*, 64, 2, 43–44.

Grove, R., Clapham, H., Moodie, T., Gurrin, S., and Hall, G. (2023). '"Living in a world that's not about us": the impact of everyday life on the health and wellbeing of autistic women and gender diverse people.' *Women's Health*, 19.

Harry-Hernandez, S., Reisner, S.L., Schrimshaw, E.W., Radix, A., *et al.* (2020). 'Gender dysphoria, mental health, and poor sleep health among transgender and gender nonbinary individuals: a qualitative study in New York City.' *Transgender Health*, 5, 1, 59–68.

Hart, E. (2023). Tweet. https://x.com/iHartEricka/status/1647650247952073216.

Haskins, N., Whitfield-Williams, M., Shillingford, M.A., Singh, A., Moxley, R., and Ofauni, C. (2013). 'The experiences of black master's counseling students: a phenomenological inquiry.' *Counselor: Education and Supervision*, 52, 3.

Hatzenbuehler, M.L., Lattanner, M.R., McKetta, A., and Pachankis, J.E. (2024). 'Structural stigma and LGBTQ+ health: a narrative review of quantitative studies.' *Lancet Public Health*, 9, 2.

Haynes, S. (2019). 'The World Health Organization will stop classifying transgender people as having a "mental disorder".' *TIME Magazine*. https://time.com/5596845/world-health-organization-transgender-identity.

Hendricks, M.L. and Testa, R.J. (2012). 'A conceptual framework for clinical work with transgender and gender nonconforming clients: an adaptation of the minority stress model.' *Professional Psychology: Research and Practice*, 43, 5, 460–467.

Hillier, A., Gallop, N., Mendes, E., Tellez, D., *et al.* (2019). 'LGBTQ+ and autism spectrum disorder: experiences and challenges.' *International Journal of Transgender Health*, 21, 1, 98–110.

Holmberg, M.H., Martin, S.G., and Lunn, M.R. (2022). 'Supporting sexual and gender minority health-care workers.' *Nature Reviews Nephrology*, 18, 339–340.

Holmes, L.G., Ames, J.L., Massolo, M.L., Nunes, D.N., and Croen, L.A. (2022). 'Improving the sexual and reproductive health and health care of autistic people.' *Pediatrics*, 149, 4.

Hope, S. (2019). *Person-Centred Counselling for Trans and Gender Diverse People: A Practical Guide*. London: Jessica Kingsley Publishers.

Horton, C. (2024). 'The Cass Review: cis-supremacy in the UK's approach to healthcare for trans children.' *International Journal of Transgender Health*, 1–25.

Human Rights Watch. (2024). 'Sudan: ethnic cleansing in West Darfur'. www.hrw.org/news/2024/05/09/sudan-ethnic-cleansing-west-darfur.

Jackson, C. (2023). 'Pride month 2023: 9% of adults identify as LGBT+.' *Ipsos*. www.ipsos.com/en/pride-month-2023-9-of-adults-identify-as-lgbt.

Jones, B.A., Haycraft, E., Murjan, S., and Arcelus, J. (2016a). 'Body dissatisfaction and disordered eating in trans people: a systematic review of the literature.' *International Review of Psychiatry*, 28, 1, 81–94.

Jones, B.A., Arcelus, J., Bouman, W.P., and Haycraft, E. (2016b). 'Sport and transgender people: a systematic review of the literature relating to sport participation and competitive sport policies.' *Sports Medicine*, 47, 4, 701–716.

Jones, F., Hamilton, J., and Kargas, N. (2024). 'Accessibility and affirmation in counselling: an exploration into neurodivergent clients' experiences.' *Counselling and Psychotherapy Research*, 25, 1.

Jones, J.M. (2022). 'LGBT identification in U.S. ticks up to 7.1%.' *Gallup*. https://news.gallup.com/poll/389792/lgbt-identification-ticks-up. aspx.

Jones, M.S. and Worthen, M.G.F. (2023). 'Measuring the prevalence and impact of adverse childhood experiences in the lives of LGBTQ individuals: a much-needed expansion.' *Child Abuse & Neglect*, 106560.

Jung, C.G. and Jaffé, A. (1963). *Memories, Dreams, Reflections*. New York: Random House.

Kaba, M. (2021.) *We Do This 'Til We Free Us: Abolitionist Organising and Transforming Justice*. London: Haymarket Books.

Kaye, H. (2023). 'The dark history of gay men, lobotomies and Walter Jackson Freeman II.' *attitude*. www.attitude.co.uk/culture/sexuality/the-dark-gay-history-of-lobotomies-and-walter-jackson-freeman-ii-419069.

Keating, L. and Muller, R.T. (2019). 'LGBTQ+ based discrimination is associated with PTSD symptoms, dissociation, emotion dysregulation, and attachment insecurity among LGBTQ+ adults who have experienced trauma.' *Journal of Trauma and Dissociation*, 12, 1, 124–141.

Khudiakova, V. and Chasteen, A.L. (2022). 'The experiences of stigmatization and discrimination in autistic people of different genders and sexualities.' *Journal of Interpersonal Relations, Intergroup Relations and Identity*, 15, 139–151.

Koch, A. (2012). *Dreams and the Person-Centered Approach: Cherishing Client Experiencing*. Monmouth: PCCS Books.

Krupnik, V. (2021). 'Tackling hyperarousal: an integrative multimodal approach.' *Cognitive Neuropsychiatry*, 26, 3, 199–212.

Lees, K. (2019). 'Sometimes trans people suck at sports (and they should be allowed to).' https://iamkatylees.com/2019/03/23/sometimes-trans-people-suck-at-sports-and-they-should-be-allowed-to.

Lefevor, G.T., Boyd-Rogers, C.C., Sprague, B.M., and Janis, R.A. (2019). 'Health disparities between genderqueer, transgender, and cisgender individuals: an extension of minority stress theory.' *Journal of Counseling Psychology*, 66, 4, 385–395.

Lewis, L.F., Ward, C., Jarvis, N., and Cawley, E. (2021). '"Straight sex is complicated enough!": the lived experiences of autistics who are gay, lesbian, bisexual, asexual, or other sexual orientations.' *Journal of Autism and Developmental Disorders*, 51, 7, 2324–2337.

Lin, L., Stamm, K., and Christidis, P. (2018). 'How diverse is the psychology workforce?' *Monitor on Psychology*, 49, 2.

Lowary, J. (2022). 'Study finds LGBQ people report higher rates of adverse childhood experiences than straight people, worse mental health as adults.' *VUMC News*. https://news.vumc.org/2022/02/24/study-finds-lgbq-people-report-higher-rates-of-adverse-childhood-experiences-than-straight-people-worse-mental-health-as-adults.

Madrigal-Borloz, V. (2023). 'End of mission statement (Country Visit to the United Kingdom of Great Britain and Northern Ireland (24 April–5 May 2023).' *United Nations*. https://digitallibrary.un.org/record/4044617?v=pdf&ln=en.

Mangen, K.H. (2023). 'OCD and scrupulosity symptoms in the LGBTQ+ community.' *Graduate Research Theses & Dissertations*, 7335.

Maslow, A. (1968). *Toward a Psychology of Being*. New York: Van Nostrand Reinhold.

McElroy, I. (2022). 'Reimagining the stories we tell about trans love.' *Elle*. www.elle.com/life-love/opinions-features/a39093298/transgender-love-relationships-lgbtq-valentines-day.

McKenzie-Mavinga, I. (2007). 'Understanding black issues in postgraduate counsellor training.' *Counselling and Psychotherapy Research*, 5, 4, 263–307.

McKinley, P.M. (2024). 'Not just Trump: America's growing problem with race.' *Just Security*. www.justsecurity.org/97409/trump-americas-problem-race.

McNeil, J., Bailey, L., Ellis, S., Morton, J., and Regan, M. (2012). *Trans Mental Health Study 2012*. www.scottishtrans.org/wp-content/uploads/2013/03/trans_mh_study.pdf.

Mearns, D. (1999). 'Person-centred therapy with configurations of the self.' *Counselling*, 10, 2, 125–130.

Mearns, D. and Thorne, B. (2000). *Person-Centred Counselling in Action*. London: SAGE.

Meckler, L., Natanson, H., and Harden, J.D. (2024). 'In states with laws targeting LGBTQ issues, school hate crimes quadrupled.' *Washington Post*. www.washingtonpost.com/education/2024/03/12/school-lgbtq-hate-crimes-incidents.

Meneguzzo, P., Zuccaretti, D., Tenconi, E., and Favaro, A. (2024). 'Transgender body image: weight dissatisfaction, objectification & identity – complex interplay explored via matched group.' *International Journal of Clinical and Health Psychology*, 24, 1.

Meyer, I.H. (2003). 'Prejudice, social stress, and mental health in lesbian, gay, and bisexual populations: conceptual issues and research evidence.' *Psychological Bulletin*, 129, 5, 674.

Moses, K. and Cole, M. (2023). 'Heteronormativity and counselor self-efficacy working with sexual and gender minority youth.' *Journal of Child and Adolescent Counseling*, 9, 3, 303–315.

Nagata, J.M., Ganson, K.T., and Austin, S.B. (2020). 'Emerging trends in eating disorders among sexual and gender minorities.' *Current Opinion in Psychiatry*, 33, 6, 562–567.

Naughton, M. and Tudor, K. (2017). 'Being white.' *Transactional Analysis Journal*, 36, 2, 159–171.

Neves, S. (2023). 'The big issue: are you GSRD competent?' *Therapy Today*, 34, 5.

Oxfam International. (2024). 'Daily death rate in Gaza higher than any other major 21st century conflict.' www.oxfam.org/en/press-releases/daily-death-rate-gaza-higher-any-other-major-21st-century-conflict-oxfam.

Panfil, V.R. (2018). 'Young and unafraid: queer criminology's unbounded potential.' *Palgrave Communications*, 4, 110.

Pappy, A. (2024). 'ICYMI: new data shows that nearly 30% of Gen Z adults identify as LGBTQ+.' *Human Rights Campaign*. www.hrc.org/press-releases/icymi-new-data-shows-that-nearly-30-of-gen-z-adults-identify-as-lgbtq.

Parker, L.L. and Harriger, J.A. (2020). 'Eating disorders and disordered eating behaviors in the LGBT population: a review of the literature. *Journal of Eating Disorders*, 8, 1, 1–20.

Parsons, V. (2020). 'Liz Truss reveals "shocking" plan to remove health-care for trans youth, slammed as an "extraordinary" attack on equality.' *PinkNews*. www.thepinknews.com/2020/04/23/liz-truss-trans-rights-gender-recognition-act-reform-healthcare-puberty-blockers-backlash.

Pritilata, M. (2022). 'Parents say trans youth were "left in limbo" following Tavistock legal case.' *Open Democracy*. www.opendemocracy.net/en/5050/mermaids-report-tavistock-keira-bell-mental-health-trans-hormones.

Reynolds, E. (2022). 'Transgender children face discrimination even at primary school level.' *British Psychological Society*. www.bps.org.uk/research-digest/transgender-children-face-discrimination-even-primary-school-level.

Rogers, C. (1957) 'The necessary and sufficient conditions of therapeutic personality change.' *Journal of Consulting Psychology*, 21, 95–103.

Roskams, M. (2023). 'The sexual orientation of usual residents aged 16 years and over in England and Wales, Census 2021 data.' Office for National Statistics. www.ons.gov.uk/peoplepopulationandcommunity/culturalidentity/sexuality/bulletins/sexualorientationenglandandwales/census2021.

Santonicollo, F. and Rollè, L. (2024). 'The role of minority stress in disordered eating: a systematic review of the literature.' *Eating and Weight Disorders*, 29, 1, 41.

Sharfman, A. and Cobb, P. (2023). 'Sexual orientation, UK: 2021 and 2022.' Office for National Statistics. www.ons.gov.uk/peoplepopulationandcommunity/culturalidentity/sexuality/bulletins/sexualidentityuk/2021and2022.

Siegel, D.J. (2010). *Mindsight: The New Science of Personal Transformation*. New York: Bantam Dell.

Siegel, D.P. (2023). 'The trans joy missing from media coverage and legislation.' *Yes! Magazine*. www.yesmagazine.org/opinion/2023/05/29/trans-joy-missing-media-coverage-legislation.

Spandler, H. and Carr, S. (2022). 'Lesbian and bisexual women's experiences of aversion therapy in England.' *History of the Human Sciences*, 35, 3–4, 218–236.

Stonewall. (2021). 'The truth about trans.' www.stonewall.org.uk/resources/lgbtq-hubs/trans-hub/the-truth-about-trans.

Strang, J.F., Kenworthy, L., Dominska, A., Sokoloff, J., *et al.* (2014). 'Increased gender variance in autism spectrum disorders and attention deficit hyperactivity disorder.' *Archives of Sexual Behaviour*, 43, 8, 1525–33.

Strudwick, P. (2011). 'Conversion therapy: she tried to make me "pray away the gay".' *The Guardian*, 27 May. www.theguardian.com/world/2011/may/27/gay-conversion-therapy-patrick-strudwick.

Thomas, T. (2024). 'Chalmers GIC pauses all gender surgery referrals for under 25s, cites Cass review.' *Trans Safety Network*. https://transsafety.network/posts/chalmers-gic-pauses-gender-surgery-referrals-under-25s-cass-review.

Toesland, F., Gross, A., and Nikolaeva, R. (2023). '"These LGBT freaks – do we have them castrated?": inside Europe's invite-only conversion therapy conference.' *Byline Times*, 12 September. https://bylinetimes.com/2023/12/09/these-lgbt-freaks-do-we-have-them-castrated-inside-europes-invite-only-conversion-therapy-conference.

Trevor Project. (2022). 'Eating disorders among LGBQ youth.' *The Trevor Project*. www.thetrevorproject.org/research-briefs/eating-disorders-among-lgbtq-youth-feb-2022.

Turban, J.L., Beckwith, N., Reisner, S.L., and Keuroghlian, A.S. (2020). 'Association between recalled exposure to gender identity conversion efforts and psychological distress and suicide attempts among transgender adults.' *JAMA Psychiatry*, 77, 1, 68–76.

Turmaud, D.R. (2021). 'The truth about therapists: Taking therapists off of the "superhuman" pedestal we put them on.' *Psychology Today*. www.psychologytoday.com/us/blog/lifting-the-veil-trauma/202106/the-truth-about-therapists.

UKCP. (2023). 'UKCP update on conversion therapy.' www.psychotherapy.org.uk/news/ukcp-update-on-conversion-therapy.

UNICEF. (2021). 'UNICEF condemns latest bout of "horrific" violence against children during armed attack on displaced people's camp in eastern DRC.' www.unicef.org/press-releases/unicef-condemns-latest-bout-horrific-violence-against-children-during-armed-attack.

VanBronkhorst, S.B., Edwards, E.M., Roberts, D.E., Kist, K., *et al.* (2021). 'Suicidality among psychiatrically hospitalized lesbian, gay, bisexual, transgender, queer, and/or questioning youth: risk and protective factors.' *LGBT Health*, 8, 6.

Villarreal, D. (2023). 'LGBTQ people are more likely to be incarcerated and face sexual violence behind bars. Here's how survivors are changing the system for the better.' *LGBTQ Nation*. www.lgbtqnation.com/2021/12/lgbtq-people-likely-incarcerated-face-sexual-violence-behind-bars-heres-survivors-changing-system-better.

Walker, N. (2021). *Neuroqueer Heresies: Notes on the Neurodiversity Paradigm, Autistic Empowerment, and Postnormal Possibilities*. Fort Worth, TX: Autonomous Press.

Wallisch, A., Boyd, B.A., Hall, J.P., Kurth, N.K., *et al.* (2023). 'Health care disparities among autistic LGBTQ+ people.' *Autism in Adulthood*, 5, 2, 165–174.

Walton, E. (2022). 'Genocide emergency: Russian aggression and genocide in Ukraine, August 2022.' *Genocide Watch*. https://web.archive.org/web/20220908171115/https://www.genocidewatch.com/single-post/country-report-ukraine-1.

Warrier, V., Greenberg, D.M., Weir, E., Buckingham, C., *et al.* (2020). 'Elevated rates of autism, other neurodevelopmental and psychiatric diagnoses, and autistic traits in transgender and gender-diverse individuals.' *Nature Communications*, 11, 3959.

Watkinson, R.E., Linfield, A., Tielemans, J., Francetic, I., and Munford, L. (2024). 'Gender-related self-reported mental health inequalities in primary care in England: a cross-sectional analysis using the GP Patient Survey.' *The Lancet Public Health*, 9, 2, 100–108.

Weir, E., Allison, C., and Baron-Cohen, S. (2021). 'The sexual health, orientation, and activity of autistic adolescents and adults.' *Autism Research*, 14, 11, 2342–2354.

White, N. (2024). 'How UK's deep rooted Islamophobia problem stoked far-right riots.' *The Independent*, 3 August. www.independent.co.uk/news/uk/home-news/uk-islamophobia-farright-riots-b2590693.html.

Witcomb, G.L., Claes, L., Bowman, W.P., Nixon, E., Motmans, J., and Arcelus, J. (2019). 'Experiences and psychological wellbeing outcomes associated with bullying in treatment-seeking transgender and gender-diverse youth.' *LGBT Health*, 6, 5.

Wren. (2021). 'Why I can never "recover" under NHS Mental Health Services.' *Psychiatry Is Driving Me Mad*. www.psychiatryisdrivingmemad.co.uk/post/why-i-can-never-recover-under-nhs-mental-health-services.

Wright, T., Candy, B., and King, M. (2018). 'Conversion therapies and access to transition-related healthcare in transgender people: a narrative systematic review.' *BMJ Open*, 8.

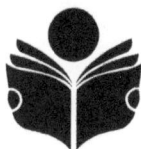

RAISING READERS
Books Build Bright Futures

Dear Reader,

We'd love your attention for one more page to tell you about the crisis in children's reading, and what we can all do.

Studies have shown that reading for fun is the **single biggest predictor of a child's future life chances** – more than family circumstance, parents' educational background or income. It improves academic results, mental health, wealth, communication skills, ambition and happiness.[1]

The number of children reading for fun is in rapid decline. Young people have a lot of competition for their time. In 2024, 1 in 10 children and young people in the UK aged 5 to 18 did not own a single book at home.[2]

Hachette works extensively with schools, libraries and literacy charities, but here are some ways we can all raise more readers:

- Reading to children for just 10 minutes a day makes a difference
- Don't give up if children aren't regular readers – there will be books for them!
- Visit bookshops and libraries to get recommendations
- Encourage them to listen to audiobooks
- Support school libraries
- Give books as gifts

There's a lot more information about how to encourage children to read on our website: **www.RaisingReaders.co.uk**

Thank you for reading.

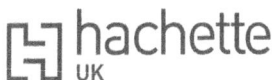

hachette
UK

---

1 National Literacy Trust, 'Book Ownership in 2024', November 2024, https://literacytrust.org.uk/research-services/research-reports/book-ownership-in-2024

2 OECD, '21st-Century Readers: Developing Literacy Skills in a Digital World', OECD Publishing, Paris, 2021, https://www.oecd.org/en/publications/21st-century-readers_a83d84cb-en.html